Nursing Issues and
Research in Terminal
Care

WILEY SERIES ON DEVELOPMENTS IN NURSING RESEARCH

Series Editor

Jenifer Wilson-Barnett
Professor and Head of Department of Nursing Studies, King's College, University of London

Volume 2
Nursing Research: Ten Studies in Patient Care
Edited by
JENIFER WILSON-BARNETT

Volume 3
Psychiatric Nursing Research
Edited by
JULIA BROOKING
Lecturer in Nursing Studies, King's College, University of London

Volume 4
Research in Preventive Community Nursing Care
Edited by
ALISON WHILE
Lecturer in Nursing Studies, King's College, University of London

Volume 5
Research in the Nursing Care of Elderly People
Edited by
PAULINE FIELDING
Director of Nursing Services, Whipps Cross Hospital, London

Volume 7 (in preparation)
Changing Perspectives in Nursing Research
Edited by
JENIFER WILSON-BARNETT AND SARAH ROBINSON*
**Research Fellow, Department of Nursing Studies, King's College, University of London*

WILEY SERIES ON
DEVELOPMENTS IN NURSING RESEARCH
VOLUME 6

Nursing Issues and Research in Terminal Care

Edited by

JENIFER WILSON-BARNETT
Professor and Head of Department of Nursing Studies, King's College, University of London, UK
and
JENNIFER RAIMAN
Education Adviser, Cancer Relief Macmillan Fund
Research Fellow, Department of Therapeutics, The London Hospital Medical College, UK

A Wiley Medical Publication

JOHN WILEY & SONS
Chichester · New York · Brisbane · Toronto · Singapore

Library of Congress Cataloging-in-Publication Data:

Nursing issues and research in terminal care/edited by Jenifer Wilson-Barnett and Jennifer Raiman.
     p. cm. — (Wiley series on developments in nursing research; v. 6)
    Includes index.
    ISBN 0 471 91795 8 (pbk.)
    1. Terminal care. 2. Terminal care — Psychological aspects.
3. Nursing — Psychological aspects. I. Wilson-Barnett, Jenifer.
II. Raiman, Jennifer. III. Series. IV. Series: Wiley medical publication.
    [DNLM: 1. Nursing Care. 2. Terminal Care. W1 WI53LF v. 6 / WY
152 N974655]
RT87.T45N9 1988
362.1′75—dc19
DNLM/DLC
for Library of Congress   87–31644 CIP

British Library Cataloguing in Publication Data:

Nursing issues and research in terminal care.
    — (Wiley series on developments in nursing research; v. 6).
    1. Terminal care 2. Nursing
    I. Wilson-Barnett, Jenifer II. Raiman, Jennifer
    610.73′61   R726.8

    ISBN 0 471 91795 8

Phototypeset by Photo·graphics, Honiton, Devon
Printed and bound in Great Britain by Anchor Brendon Ltd, Tiptree, Essex

All contributors to this book have been associated with Cancer Relief Macmillan Fund.

Researchers and practitioners depend on each other, and some of the products of this partnership are reflected in the book.

Contents

Part 5: Comfort Care

Part 6: Coordination of Care

Part 7: Conclusion

List of Contributors

FRANCES FOTHERGILL BOURBONNAIS, Associate Professor, School of Nursing, University of Ottawa, Canada

JUDITH HILL, Regional Nurse, Continuing Care, Wessex Regional Health Authority, UK

ANN NASH, The Dorothy House Foundation, Macmillan Service, Bath, UK

JENNIFER RAIMAN, Department of Pharmacology and Therapeutics, The London Hospital Medical College, London, UK

SALLY SIMS, Catholic College of Education, Sydney, Australia

MARY THOMAS, Strathcarron Hospice, Scotland, UK

ALISON WHILE, Department of Nursing Studies, King's College, London, UK

JENIFER WILSON-BARNETT, Department of Nursing Studies, King's College, London, UK

Series Preface

Developments in Nursing Research

Nursing science is derived from an integration of knowledge in other disciplines and from original nursing research studies. As more relevant research is completed key areas are developing, benefiting from different approaches in various patient care settings. The purpose of this series is to publish literature reviews and original material in such areas to promote nursing progress and knowledge.

Preface

Nursing Issues and Research in Terminal Care

This volume reviews issues of importance to nursing care of those with terminal illness. From social aspects, to family care and symptom relief, authors have attempted to review research in this area. They have utilized findings from other disciplines, as well as describing nursing studies. Suggestions for future research have also been made.

As with other volumes in this series, editors have not attempted to introduce a uniform style throughout the text. Indeed, one of the most interesting features tends to be the variety of emphasis and rich mixture of contributions. Many new developments in terminal care have been discussed and the central role of the nurse is clearly evident from all this work.

Part 1 Introduction

Nursing Issues and Research in Terminal Care
Edited by J. Wilson-Barnett and J. Raiman
© 1988 John Wiley & Sons Ltd.

CHAPTER 1

Key Areas for Terminal Care* Nursing

JENIFER WILSON-BARNETT

Caring for a dying person and his family extends all the fundamental skills a nurse should have. The sensitivities, knowledge and practical abilities necessary can only be developed over the years but those who are cared for rightly expect every nurse to have all these attributes. Even for those who are acknowledged experts it is the mark of a true professional to question one's performance and constantly evaluate how fully the client's needs are fulfilled. Despite evidence that better care is being provided, that fewer needs remain unmet and more specially trained staff exist, many nurses are aware that their own knowledge can always be improved. New approaches which reflect changes in society should be considered, and innovations in medical care must be examined for their influences on other carers. This constantly changing situation is reflected by the keen interest and fine example set by health care teams and specialists caring for the terminally ill. The recent spate of reports evaluating services and supporting these developments demonstrates that such staff combine a scientific appraisal of what has been achieved with a drive to promote real caring for those most in need. Nurses too are in the forefront of this progress and their own endeavours to provide a reliable knowledge base for their practice led to this book.

Aimed to review knowledge within this area of terminal care nursing, this book also critically examines nursing interventions which should

---

* 'By terminal care is meant the treatment of patients, primarily cancer sufferers, for whom the advent of death is diagnosed as being imminent and therefore the emphasis is no longer curative but palliative in nature.' Hedley Taylor (1983), p. 6.

(or should not) be provided for patients and suggests specific areas where research is needed. By describing what services are provided and what patients and their relatives say about these, our hope is to help all those nurses who care for the dying to become more sensitive to their needs.

Nurses do have a unique contribution to make and special responsibilities which they sometimes share with others in the team. More understanding of these may help to promote excellence in care and orient the reader to our background philosophy of terminal care. Structure will be provided by five key functions of nursing described on a previous occasion (Wilson-Barnett, 1983) as these will also show how the essence of terminal care draws from that care which should be known as 'nursing'.

The first nursing function is:

To understand illness and treatment from the patient's viewpoint and situation.

Different cultural and social backgrounds affect how people experience their life, illness, and finally the terminal phase of their life. Expectations, preferences, opinions and values determine their responses to illness and treatment. As Pilowski (1975) says:

illness is the patients' experience . . . and no two patients experience the same illness in the same way. Why therefore should their care be identical?

Despite sociological analysis of illness behaviour, which attempts to draw common themes from many diverse responses, it is clear that patients and their families each have a quite particular set of views. The context for care and the combined influence of the family in determining priorities must be understood in order to provide relevant care. Nurses therefore need to understand the social setting and family if they are to plan and set shared goals.

Cultural and religious norms and expectations of the rituals and behaviour associated with dying vary. Usual customs in relation to the degree of family involvement with care of a dying member, the extent to which death is a taboo subject and the associated beliefs all affect the type of role a nurse adopts. Unless this is assessed sensitively, inappropriate interventions might be proffered.

Participation in care by patients and family members may be appreciated, even assumed, or this may not be possible or taken on unwillingly. Gauging whether 'control' and 'a partnership' in care is beneficial, required for some or all, is important. Despite evidence that this is therapeutic in some settings as witnessed by research reviewed in the CURN project (CURN, 1982), it may not be indicated at the stage when death is imminent for some patients. Their socialization and social mores as well as their physical strength determines this. However, experts in the field of palliative care agree that the patient and his family in the community ideally lead the health care team (Charles-Edwards, 1986). Lunt and Jenkins' (1983) useful papers on goal-setting in terminal care clearly demonstrate that staff appreciate this process. As they become more competent and confident it seems a natural extension to include patients and their families in this activity. The extent to which this is undertaken by nurses varies, and Lunt's team (Lunt, 1985) did not find significant improvements in this orientation to care in specialized hospices over a three-year study period.

In the terminal care setting, where a continuous relationship with staff should be possible, such decisions as where the patient dies and when he requires hospital or hospice care as an inpatient or for daycare are frequently necessary. Ultimately the decision must be based on a comprehensive appraisal of the social and family background. Continuous support for the family after the patient has died is also clearly a nursing responsibility. Bereavement counselling becomes so much more meaningful if a good relationship has been established beforehand and the nurse knows how the family has coped and whether terminal care met their expectations.

Family care is obviously an important area of 'terminal nursing'. However, Hinds' (1985) work in Canada shows that many families have unfulfilled needs for information and support. One-third of the 83 families studied coped badly, needing more help with physical care, but the most commonly cited need was someone with whom to discuss their fears. (Further insights into the North American terminal care scene are provided in this book by Frances Fothergill Bourbonnais in Chapter 2.) Lack of support was also found to be a dominant concern for a sample of spouses and family in the United States. Lewis's 1986 review of studies concluded that families needed more information on methods of giving care and emergency measures and more emotional help for the patients and themselves. Spiritual needs were also

unfulfilled. Signs of distress and psychological morbidity among family
members were found to be very common in these studies.

Bereavement counselling (discussed by Judith Hill — Chapter 3), as
devised by Dracup and Breu (1978), is frequently needed and Macmillan
nurses see this as a vital part of continuing care. This is clearly
facilitated by understanding the needs of those who are grieving.
Dracup and Breu (1978) identify the goals for this type of support, as:

1. to be with the dying person
2. to be helpful to the dying person
3. to be assured of the comfort of the patient
4. to be informed of the patient's condition
5. to be informed of impending death
6. to ventilate emotions
7. to have comfort and support for the family
8. to be accepted, supported and comforted by the health professionals.

Thus care must be planned to meet the needs of the family as well
as the patient. In turn, his needs will also be more fulfilled by stronger,
more supportive relatives. No one should be nursed in isolation, but
always by exploiting a social network.

A related function for nursing is:

the provision of continuous psychological care during illness or
critical events.

There is now realization by nurses that this area of care is vital to
patients yet relatively poorly carried out in many settings. Evidence
that general nurses would give greater importance to this 'if they had
time' exists (Hockey, 1978). Yet physical care is still given a priority
in many areas. Supposedly inadequate preparation and skills are
responsible, yet where psychological interventions are given by nurses
clearly beneficial results are obtained (Wilson-Barnett, 1984).

In terminal care knowledge of psychological reactions and expertise
is essential to inform, support and comfort the patient. Adjustment to
the realization that death is imminent, avoiding persistent denial,
anxiety or depression, is desirable. Open communication and sensitive
reactions to the patient and his loved ones by staff is essential to help
in achieving this aim. Change in the philosophy of care over the last

decade has led to a much greater awareness by nurses that they should engage in this aspect of practice. Reports by Bond (1978) and Knight and Field (1981) documenting unclear, unhelpful or confused patterns of communication in terminal care settings helped to provide a further impetus to improve. More recently Field (1984) found that nurses in more general settings were expressing more constructive and knowledgeable suggestions for providing psychological care for those who were dying. Consistent responses from a delphi survey (Hitch and Murgatroyd, 1983) on British nurses' views of terminal care also demonstrated that many acknowledge the importance of psychological care but feel they lack sufficient preparation. Counselling skills may be considered more suitable for specialized and advanced training, but those who continually work with the dying and their families, as the Macmillan nurses do, need to feel confident in this aspect of care. Courses are run by many institutions and not only does this clearly help clients but nurses too can also learn to cope with the pressure of this type of involvement. Considerations of potential burnout and withdrawal from these stresses has led to suggestions that nurses should rotate through specialities and not remain in one area of care (Maguire, 1985). Some may well feel this is appropriate. Opportunities should perhaps be offered but not instituted in a blanket way unnecessarily. With adequate training nurses themselves should be more empowered to assess their own health and be accountable for providing support to each other as part of their professional life.

However, the maturity and the skills necessary to engage in this work cannot be underestimated. As Sally Sims discusses in Chapter 5, individual and changing reactions to the process of dying must be faced and accepted. It is this very element of 'personal care' which is so fundamental to terminal care.

Without the skill to communicate empathy, understanding and reassurance, a nurse will not be able to give adequate psychological care (Macleod Clark, 1983). This set of professional skills has to be learnt through careful feedback and rehearsal. Greater educational opportunity and more experience in terminal care tends to be associated with greater understanding and skill (Reisetter and Thomas, 1986). Preparation necessary to fulfil this function usually contains theoretical, classroom activities and supervised practice. Video feedback and role play is said to be particularly useful in gaining insight into one's own communication behaviour (Maguire, 1985).

Psychological care for the dying must be based on a confident and comfortable understanding of what death means for the carer. Attitudes to death are frequently bound up in social taboos and discussion of fears and beliefs is usually helpful for nurses who enter this arena. Several studies have evaluated fairly modest educational inputs for their effects on nurses' attitudes to dying and related anxiety. Consistently researchers such as Ross (1978) and Laube (1977) demonstrate that considering and sharing personal attitudes and fears with others in an experimental workshop helps to strengthen nurses' coping when faced with death. Avoidance patterns and reduced levels of care for those who are dying are unforgivable and only when staff learn to feel comfortable themselves will patients really 'open up' and trust them. Evidence that nurses are reluctant and uneasy is plentiful. From America, Keck and Walther (1977) found that nurses did not spend longer in giving psychological care to those designated as dying and often distressed, than to other patients on a general ward. Blocking tactics and closed communication styles are also found within many health professional groups. Maguire's (1985) work with communication workshops demonstrates the continuing need for this type of opportunity for them in training and repeatedly throughout their professional life.

Many studies now confirm that continuous work within a progressive organization devoted to the care of the dying facilitates the much needed psychological and spiritual care. Beliefs and faith are certainly more important to patients at the end of their life, just as at any other stressful time. Ready comfort and attention from clergy and a true appreciation of the significance of spiritual support are more evident in specialized hospice care. Reports from relatives in a retrospective comparative study by Parkes (1978) also showed that information needs were satisfactory and support was always forthcoming, when needed, for those cared for by a home-centred or hospice team rather than a general hospital staff. Lunt's (1985) work confirms this, both patients and relatives expressing much more satisfaction when experiencing hospice care. Others were less likely to talk to nurses about their concerns. In hospices the last 24 hours of care was more likely to be aimed at family care, whereas a third of relatives had poor or mixed memories of this phase when patients died in hospital.

Indeed, this is supported by the work of Bowling and Cartwright (1982) from a national survey of death and bereavement among the elderly. The vast majority (74 per cent) of people who died in hospital did so alone without relatives or friends present, but this was the case for only a minority (15 per cent) of those who died at home. This is an alarming finding given that the most common fear expressed by those anticipating death is of dying alone, and that two-thirds of those who die do so in hospital.

Lunt's research team concludes (Paper C, p. 24), 'The consistency of findings suggests that views reported are based on real differences in the behaviour and approach of hospice and district general hospital staff, and indicate practical ways in which improvements might be sought'. Throughout this book such implications will, we hope, become clear.

The third area of care is most complex and often poorly understood.

Nurses help patients to cope with illness or potential health problems, whether this be mental or physical coping, patients need guidance to reduce discomfort, information to think about their problems, to plan their actions and strategies and other resources to aid independence and adjustment.

All the elements usually conceived as stressful, threat, loss and challenge, are relevant to those who are suffering from a terminal illness. If extreme stress persists without adequate coping, further physical and psychological harm may occur. By aiding adjustment or coping and providing a supportive buffer to the effects of stress nurses can be an invaluable resource. Ultimately it is the patient and his spouse or family who adjust, make plans and support each other, but they sometimes need facilitation and practical help. Good social and psychological care enables a majority of people to adjust to their loss.

Coping with physical and domestic problems becomes exceedingly difficult with progressive weakness and symptoms. Despite ingenious solutions to avoid lifting or manage stairs, coping ability may be destroyed by distressing or embarrassing symptoms. Pain control has advanced significantly in the last decade, since the start of the hospice movement. Official reports on terminal care (Standing Medical Advisory Committee, 1980; Council of Europe, 1981) all advise that regimes adopted to treat pain prophylactically by regular, adequate analgesia to avoid breakthrough pain maintain a better quality of life and permit adequate coping with changes in life circumstances.

Symptoms such as pain, nausea, anorexia, constipation, dry mouth, insomnia, dyspnoea, vomiting, oedema and cough were reported by a group of terminally ill patients and ranked in that order of frequency by Twycross (1986). These must all be attended to medically but nurses can have a vital function in helping to reduce associated suffering and facilitate coping by useful practical tips. Foods, drinks, room temperature and physical activity may affect all these symptoms. Hints from other patients to cope with these can be passed on to others currently in need. Molly Parsons, Mary Thomas, and Jennifer Raiman explore some of these problems in Chapters 6 and 7.

Evidence that specialists in terminal care manage to alleviate associated symptoms has been produced in both comparative studies (Lunt, 1985) and retrospective analysis (Parkes, 1978). However, these reports also provide data on neglect for those who die unattended at home and for those in hospitals, who have a greater chance of becoming confused and overmedicated.

Coping is reliant on information for making realistic plans and the opportunity to think and talk through ways of managing the present and the future. Research which explores the efficacy of contact and support for patients from other fellow sufferers is directly relevant to this. Van den Borne, Pruyn and van den Heuvel (1987) found that such contacts were most useful if discussion was based on a clear understanding of the condition and when professionally given information was originally satisfactory. Support groups can be most helpful for patients and families. These are sometimes run by hospice teams or organized by voluntary organizations. Successful copers can often help others by example and suggestion and spouses report enormous relief in being able to share fears and worries. The current trend to advocate more daycare facilities from the hospice base (Wilkes, 1980) could include groups as one of the events of the day.

Guidance with and provision of aides and equipment is essential for those coping with terminal care at home. Commodes, laundry services and dressings or absorbent materials should all be available, and as Charles-Edwards (1986) explains, these really can have a great impact on the lives of those who need them. After this families are usually much more able to cope with difficulties in basic care.

District nurses and those constantly caring for the dying or grieving, such as the Macmillan nursing teams, have accumulated practical wisdom related to the next core nursing function: 'to provide comfort'. Although this may be included in aspects of psychological care and symptom relief it infers more. It really consists of additional and extra components of nursing which provide excellence or sensitivity. High-quality service in any walk of life is based on willingness, thoughtfulness and charm. In nursing it also combines skill to assess what attention may bring comfort. Sally Sims' review of complementary approaches to care in Chapter 8 introduces less well tested, but clearly needed, interventions. In an open-minded approach to the art of nursing we must learn to evaluate all possible means of providing comfort.

Extra niceties, but also basic comprehensive care, can provide comfort. A warm bath, clean sheets, moisturizing lotions and scented pillows, relaxation, music and body massage, can all be included. Personal items of significance for someone who is dying should be highly prized and recognized. Letters, photographs and pets can all bring comfort and should be easily accessible.

Fatigue and restlessness are frequently experienced by those who are bedfast. Lack of stimulation or diversion is often responsible and frequently means a nursing challenge. Poor concentration, though, may also rule out previous forms of enjoyment such as reading or watching television. However, a planned day provides variety and structure and incorporates periods of activity and rest. This helps to prevent a feeling of helplessness and boredom, particularly if each day holds something different. Clearly this can be included as part of comfort care.

Use of massage could be so much more widespread. However, Sally Sims' (1986) study shows its introduction has to be carefully planned to promote understanding of the purpose. Benefits of feeling more relaxed and 'cared for' should not be underestimated. This opportunity to provide a pleasant and straightforward comfort measure should be taken by many more staff. Other treatments provided in beauty salons may also be really appreciated by patients. For instance, facial and hand treatments may be used to spend a relaxing period which may lead to more open communication and boost morale. Family members may also enjoy giving such comforts and should be helped to master such techniques where possible.

Lastly, coordination of care is seen as a central nursing function:

> Nurses should act as coordinators of treatments and other events affecting a patient. They should help others in providing treatments and monitor the responses of the patients to prevent harmful effects.

Continuous assessment of symptoms and responses to treatment and knowledge of what each professional can contribute to care are essential for this function. Liaison with members of a health care team can lead to constructive collaborative actions and fewer frustrating delays in treatment. However, the nurse's responsibility to provide comprehensive, holistic care frequently puts her into the position of being a primary source of care and referral. This therefore means that it is her job to involve others and encourage their further commitment.

Negotiation and diplomatic skills are needed in terminal care as with every other area of health service. Expertise in clinical care, diligence and first-hand knowledge of a family should ensure that other professionals attend to the requests of nurses, as explained in Chapters 4 and 9. Despite anecdotal complaints to/from all members of the team at times, multidisciplinary education, particularly advanced in the field of terminal care (Wilkes, 1980), makes this aspect of work less stressful.

However, working within the community and representing the wishes of families to others widens the role of the nurse. Opinions and values adopted and expressed by the general public can be influenced by professional views. Behaviour which indicates that friends and acquaintances of a dying person are apprehensive and estranged is distressing. Yet work of the terminal care movement within and through special teams is having a noticeable effect on people's ability to talk about death, as Rees's (1982) report suggests.

Throughout the spectrum of these nursing functions all aspects are relevant to the care of the dying patient and his family. This is an area where great progress has been made through social forces, concerted efforts by charities and individuals. However, there is still a tremendous amount to be done, not least in promoting good nursing practice, based on a sound education and research.

Hence these five key areas provide a structure for this book of independent chapters. Chapter 2 by Frances Fothergill Bourbonnais, Terminal Care: A Canadian Perspective, shows that cultural or *societal* influences have a bearing on how terminal care services and nursing develop. It is interesting that there are similarities and differences with the British system. The editors considered it more worthwhile to devote pages to this less familiar context for care than review the British scene, which has already been done proficiently (Taylor, 1983).

Bereavement care and *psychological* reactions in children are reviewed by Judith Hill and Alison While respectively. It is clear from these contributions that much research has been done in these areas which provides confident guidelines for practice.

Coping with dying and distressing symptoms reflects the broad responsibility which nurses undertake in order to facilitate these processes. Deeply complex psychological reactions to dying are discussed by Sally Sims in the context of a vast area of literature only a small proportion of which has been produced by nurses, whereas Molly Parsons and Mary Thomas review several physical problems and tend to draw on a wide range of biological and medical knowledge. Nursing research has only just started to provide guidelines for practice and the mixture of clinical advice and research which produce the rationale for care in this section is impressive. The 'symptoms' chapter is perhaps directed to the nurse and the patient who are coping with distressing symptoms. Some aspects, such as mouth and wound care, have obviously been the focus of more research than other applied areas, such as sleep disturbance and fatigue.

Closely linked with alleviation of symptoms is Jennifer Raiman's chapter on pain and its management in the section on providing *comfort*. This explains these authors' adherence to the defined stages of theoretical overview assessment, intervention and evaluation. Chapter 7 and the preceding one reflect so much of importance to physical nursing care that it is unsurprising that they contain so many tables and more pages than others! The second chapter subsumed under 'comfort' care, by Sally Sims, demonstrates that new areas of nursing are in need of more systematic research, not only to provide evidence of value but to make them professionally acceptable.

Finally, the chapter on the role of the nurse in family support, by Ann Nash, provides a professional view of what is needed and valued in terminal care. Although many aspects are reviewed, *coordination* of the family's and others' contributions is really emphasized.

Despite the different orientation of all authors, clear messages are expressed on the need to do more for patients and their families and evaluate what is provided. Research is emerging, but needs to be prioritized and funded. The final chapter therefore aims to offer a few ideas for consideration.

This book may expose many areas which are difficult to both study and manage in the clinical setting. For this reason the concluding section reviews further needs for research. Patients' and families' experiences should determine areas of practice, research and nursing education. Each aspect should benefit from the other, although it seems at times that the most essential functions are the least subject to research and perhaps never can be. Without attempting to review the state of our science and art nursing will not progress. Each chapter is designed to be informative and questioning; if the research base does not seem obvious, it needs to be created. Those in terminal care are the ones most able to decide what studies should be done and perhaps they may also be encouraged by our suggestions.

We hope that nurses will enjoy this book, which emulates the first in this series in containing more reviews of work and less presentation of new studies. Let us hope that in a few years more projects will be available for publication and improved practice.

References

Bond, S. (1978) Process of communication about cancer in a radiotherapy department, Unpublished PhD thesis, University of Edinburgh.

Bowling, A., and Cartwright, A. (1982) *Life after Death: A Study with the Elderly Widowed*. Tavistock, London.

Charles-Edwards, A. (1986) Nursing care at home. In Spilling, R. (ed.) *Terminal Care at Home*. Oxford Medical Publications, Oxford, pp. 62–68.

Council of Europe (1981) *Problems Related to Death: Care for the Dying. Final Report*.

CURN (1982) *Mutual Goal Setting in Patient Care*. Michigan Nurses Association. Grune and Stratton, New York.

Dracup, K.A., and Breu, C.S. (1978) Using nursing research findings to meet the needs of grieving spouses, *Nursing Research*, **27** (4), 212–216.

Field, D.G. (1984) 'We didn't want him to die on his own' — nurses' account of nursing dying patients, *Journal of Advanced Nursing*, **9**, 59–70.

Field, D., and Kitson, C. (1986) Formal teaching about death and dying. UK Nursing Schools, *Nursing Education Today*, **6**, 270–276.

Hinds, C. (1985) The needs of families who care for patients with cancer at home: Are we meeting them? *Journal of Advanced Nursing*, **10**, 575–581.

Hitch, P.J., and Murgatroyd, D. (1983) Professional communications in cancer care, *Journal of Advanced Nursing*, **8**, 494–505; A Delphi survey of hospital nurses, **8**, 413–422.

Hockey, L. (1978) *Woman in Nursing*. Churchill Livingstone, Edinburgh.

Keck, V.E., and Walther, L.S. (1977) Nurse encounters with dying and undying patients, *Nursing Research*, **26**(6), 465–469.

Knight, M., and Field, D. (1981) A silent conspiracy: Coping with dying cancer patients on an acute surgical ward, *Journal in Advanced Nursing*, **6**, 221–229.

Laube, J. (1977) Death and dying workshop for nurses: Its effect on their death anxiety level, *International Journal of Nursing Studies*, **14**, 111–120.

Lunt, B. (1985) A comparison of hospice and hospital care for terminally ill cancer patients and their families, Final Report, Southampton University.

Lunt, B., and Jenkins, J. (1983) Goal setting in terminal care: A method of recording treatment aims and priorities, *Journal of Advanced Nursing*, **8**, 495–505.

Macleod Clark, J. (1983) Nurse–patient communication — an analysis of conversations from surgical wards. In Wilson-Barnett, J. (ed.) *Nursing Research: Ten Studies in Patient Care*. Wiley, Chichester.

Maguire, P. (1985) Barriers to psychological care of the dying, *British Medical Journal*, **291**, 1711–1713.

Parkes, C.M. (1978) Home or hospital? Terminal care as seen by surviving spouses, *Journal of Royal College of General Practitioners*, January, 13–30.

Pilowski, I. (1975) Dimensions of abnormal illness behaviour, *Australian and New Zealand Journal of Psychiatry*, **9**, 141–147.

Rees, W.D. (1982) Role of the hospice in the care of the dying, *British Medical Journal*, **285**, 1766–1768.

Reisetter, K.H., and Thomas, B. (1986) Nursing care of the dying: Its relationship to selected nursing characteristics, *International Journal of Nursing Studies*, **23** (1), 39–50.

Ross, C.W. (1978) Nurses' personal death concerns and responses to dying patients' statements, *Nursing Research*, **27** (1), 64–68.

Simms, M. (1984) *Nurse Training for Terminal Care: A Pilot Study*. Institute for Social Science in Medical Care, London.

Sims, S. (1986) The effects of slow stroke back massage in the perceived wellbeing of female patients receiving radiotherapy for cancer, MSc, King's College, London University.

Standing Medical Advisory Committee (1980) *Terminal Care*, March.

Taylor, H. (1983) *The Hospice Movement in Britain: Its Role and its Future*. Centre for Policy on Ageing, London.

Twycross, R. (1986) Hospice Care. In Spilling, R. (ed.) *Terminal Care at Home*. Oxford Medical Publications, Oxford, pp. 96–112.

Van den Borne, H.W., Pruyn, J.F.A., and van den Heuvel, J.W.A. (1987) Effects of contacts between cancer patients on their psychological problems, *Patients Education and Counselling*, **9**, 33–51.

Wilkes, E. (1980) Terminal care: How can we do better? *Journal of Royal College of Physicians*, **20** (3), 216–218.

Wilson-Barnett, J. (1983) Key functions in nursing. The Winifred Raphael Memorial lecture, RCN, London.

Wilson-Barnett, J. (1984) Alleviating stress for hospitalized patients, *International Review of Applied Psychology*, **33**, 493–503.

Part 2   The Social Context of Care

Nursing Issues and Research in Terminal Care
Edited by J. Wilson-Barnett and J. Raiman
© 1988 John Wiley & Sons Ltd.

CHAPTER 2

Terminal Care: A Canadian Perspective

FRANCES FOTHERGILL BOURBONNAIS

The development of terminal care in Canada has followed the trend of adapting the hospice model of the United Kingdom within the structure of an active treatment hospital, namely, a palliative care unit or a palliative care service.

The Department of National Health and Welfare for Canada formed a working group to establish guidelines for the development of palliative care in Canada. The actual delivery of health care in Canada, however, is a provincial responsibility and each province is developing programs that will best meet the needs of their particular province.

Canada now has a Palliative Care Foundation* with headquarters in Toronto. There is also the *Journal of Palliative Care* published biannually for the Palliative Care Foundation by the University of Toronto Press. National Palliative Care Conferences began in 1985 to examine national issues. The most recent conference of this nature took place in Ottawa, Ontario in October 1987.

The Palliative Care Unit

Palliative care is the term commonly used for hospice care in Canada. French and English are the two official languages in Canada and the term palliative was chosen in part to prevent misinterpretation of the term hospice in the French language (Scott, 1981). The Royal Victoria Palliative Care Unit in Montreal, Quebec was the first comprehensive

---

* The Palliative Care Foundation closed its operations as from November 1987.

hospital-based hospice service. Dr Balfour Mount, who was responsible for much of the beginning of palliative care in Canada, established this unit, formerly a surgical ward, in January 1975. Today there is a palliative care centre at the Royal Victoria Hospital which has as its mandate to meet the physical, psychological, social and spiritual needs of terminally ill patients and their families. This centre consists of (1) the palliative care unit, (2) a hospital-based home care program, (3) an outpatient clinic, (4) consultation service to other parts of the hospital, (5) a bereavement follow-up service. The multidisciplinary team consists of physicians, nurses, volunteers, social worker, physiotherapist, music therapist, chaplain and psychiatrist. With a strong emphasis on research and education, this centre has become a model for terminal care in Canada (Scott, 1981).

The Palliative Care Services

This approach to palliative care consists of an interdisciplinary or multidisciplinary team which assesses terminal patients wherever they may be in the hospital setting, gives advice on symptom control, and supports families and staff as well as the patients. There is great variation in how this service is conducted. Nurses are frequently the coordinators of the services. The other team members such as social workers and dieticians may be employed part-time on this team while maintaining the remainder of their position in other departments. Other palliative care services consist of team members who devote a few hours per week to provide consultation but these same people would have full-time positions in other areas.

The term 'hospice' is also used whether this specialized resource is a free-standing structure with beds or a network of community services or a combination of central facility and home services (Cousens, Andrewes and Dean, 1987). For example, Hospice King outside of Toronto, Ontario is a palliative care service in the community with links to the Victorian Order of Nurses, who provide nursing care in the home, and links to the home care program. Thus, different organizational approaches towards palliative care have emerged. Whatever the organizational structure, Canada's development of palliative care follows the basic principles of hospice care established in the United Kingdom, that is, holistic caring, skilled health team care for effective pain and other symptom control, continual assessment of the patient's physical, psychological and spiritual needs and family involvement (Manning, 1984). The focus is on continuity of care for both patient and family.

The next section of this chapter will focus on different regions within different provinces and the approaches they have used to meet the needs for palliative care.

Palliative Care — Specific Examples

La Maison Michel Sarrazin

La Maison Michel Sarrazin in Quebec City of the province of Quebec is a comprehensive centre which includes a fifteen-bed nursing home, a close network with home care as well as hospital services and a research and training centre (Dionne and staff, 1986). It is a free-standing structure which collaborates functionally and financially with fourteen community and university affiliated hospitals as well as the local university (Laval) and its faculty. The home care service promotes dying at home whenever possible. This service began in 1983, before the inpatient facility was built in 1985. Historically, the choice in favour of a separate unit was based on the special characteristics of the Quebec region and its health care services. Quebec City, the capital of the province, has a population of half a million people and is predominantly French-speaking. It was recognized that La Maison Michel Sarrazin would be the only separate institution in the region and that the centre would be a teaching unit (Dionne and staff, 1986). In 1981, Dr Therese Vanier from St Christopher's Hospice in Sydenham was invited to Quebec City. The sharing of Dr Vanier's experiences helped to seal the commitment to develop the centre. Today La Maison Michel Sarrazin is recognized as a teaching unit in the domain of care of the dying patient. Studies are received from all the health science disciplines. As well, staff have provided teaching programs in hospitals, sessions for general practitioners and a course for volunteers. Involvement of university faculty in research and teaching activities is facilitated through an agreement between the centre and the university (Dionne and staff, 1986).

The Ottawa–Carleton Regional Palliative Care Association

The author's home region will be used to illustrate how one region developed its program. In 1979, the Ottawa–Carleton District Health Council formed a committee to develop a plan for the delivery of palliative care in that region. By 1982, the Riverside Hospital and the Ottawa Civic Hospital had developed palliative care services for their patients. Also in 1982, the Sisters of Charity together with the Canadian Cancer Society contributed a total of over one million dollars to construct a 25-bed palliative care unit in the Elisabeth Bruyere Health Centre. The Ministry of Health strongly supported the initiation of a regional program to coordinate existing services. The projected needs were the 25-bed unit, home palliative care for over 100 patients and the development of specific facilities at all acute and chronic hospitals in the region.

The current Ottawa–Carleton Regional Palliative Care Association is composed of a network of institutional and community agency service providers. The purpose of the association is to promote high-quality palliative care services in the various health care settings (hospitals and community) to coordinate aspects of palliative care provided in the region and to enhance the continuity of care provided to terminally ill patients and their families (Ottawa Report, 1986). The structure of the association comprises a Council and four standing committees: (1) the interdisciplinary professional, (2) the volunteer, (3) public relations, (4) research and education. Several subcommittees have also been established to meet the needs of patients and health professionals. For example, the patient tracking system subcommittee has been formed to plan and develop a coordinated patient tracking information system to ensure continuity of care for patients entering into the program at any level. The research subcommittee is focusing on identifying how the regional palliative care program can facilitate palliative care research. The mandate of the education subcommittee is to promote education for health professionals providing or planning to provide palliative care. Members on this committee are from the health science education institutions and the service agencies. The interdisciplinary professional committee now has subcommittees for each professional body represented, such as the nursing subcommittee.

Currently, many palliative care programs are developing on their own, which means they must compete for funds from hospital budgets and rely on fund-raising and private donations. Both in the United Kingdom and in Canada, hospice/palliative care would have had difficulty developing without the support of interested health professionals and volunteers and financial support from corporations and other forms of fund-raising.

A country the size of Canada has vast regional differences and thus palliative care programs which are developing must meet the needs specific to the different areas. For example, in St John's, the capital city of Newfoundland, Canada's most easterly province, there is a palliative care unit at the St Clare's Mercy Hospital. Newfoundland is a large but sparsely populated province, and thus patients admitted to this unit could be from many outlying regions. There is also an active home care program and, as with many British hospices, the patient is assured a bed in the unit when required (Manning, 1984).

Community-Based Palliative Care

Many family members would care for a dying relative at home if the necessary resources were available, if they were made aware of existing services and how to access them and if they were taught certain treatment and care functions. It is not feasible to tell people to care for dying relatives at home without providing the necessary support services. Patients and their families should not have to make a choice between good home care and good hospital care; both services are needed (Parkes, 1985).

The Macmillan home care nurses in the United Kingdom provide services to the terminally ill and their families at home. Two examples of community care in Canada will now be presented.

The Ottawa–Carleton Regional Palliative Care Home Care Program

Currently this program consists of a community supervisor, three palliative home care coordinators and a 25-member palliative care team of the Victorian Order of Nurses. Once a patient is admitted to the palliative home care program, one of the coordinators visits the patient and family, does an initial assessment and identifies all the services they will require to promote optimum quality for the patient's life. These services might include, for example, occupational therapy or physiotherapy. If specific nursing care is required the Victorian Order of Nurses team, prepared in palliative care, would visit the patient. Volunteers also provide assistance to patients cared for at home. Palliative care in the community must also confront the dilemma of patients with little family support. To meet this problem, one of the Anglican churches will be planning and building in the Ottawa–Carleton region a hospice to care for patients who lack support.

A major issue confronting the community-based palliative care in Ontario is that of 'shift care funding'. The phrase 'shift care' refers to the provision of nursing/attendant care for eight or more consecutive hours per day (Stephenson-Cino *et al.*, 1987). Shift care nursing is frequently an essential part of palliative planning for patients who wish to die at home. However, at this moment there is no fixed funding for professional nursing on a shift basis. There are increasing numbers of patients who wish to remain at home. Many of these patients have complex medical problems for which care must be provided (Stephenson-Cino et al., 1987). A retrospective study was done in the Hamilton–Wentworth region of Ontario to estimate the impact that lack of funding for shift care would have on the delivery of health care to palliative patients. It concluded that up to 25 per cent of patients who required shift care, but who would not have private financial resources to pay for this service, might be forced to enter hospital (Stephenson-Cino et al., 1987). Thus, the choice is removed from these patients as to whether they will die in hospital or at home. This shift care nursing also affords families some periods of rest from care as the patient approaches the final days of his/her life. Without this support, families at the end are often on the brink of exhaustion. Research is needed to clarify the effect of this family exhaustion on the bereavement process.

The Palliative Home Care Program of Calgary, Alberta

Alberta is one of Canada's most westerly provinces and Calgary is one of its major cities. The Palliative Home Care Service began in Calgary in 1980. It was the result of planning by a committee consisting of representatives from hospitals, service agencies, and the community at large (Cook Gotay, 1984). This palliative home care service was one of the first attempts in North America to provide comprehensive services for terminally ill individuals encompassing an entire city and all its hospitals. Also in the city is Hospice Calgary, a comprehensive city-wide program for palliative care. The palliative home care program is a subprogram of the overall home care program and most services are contracted for through existing agencies. The following are just a few of the many features of this program: structured support and communication systems, volunteers as an integral part of the interdisciplinary team, 24 hours per day service for seven days a week, physician-directed interdisciplinary care, and ongoing evaluation. In regard to this latter feature, three consecutive evaluative studies have been produced examining the palliative home care service from 1982 to 1984. The questions that guided the research were: what kinds of patients, families and staff were involved in the service; how was the service conducted; and what were the outcomes of the service (Cook

Gotay, 1984). Some of the highlights of the study results are as follows: the high satisfaction of patient and family with the service both at the time of receiving home care and subsequently one year later; the importance of psychosocial care to patients and families; and an increase over time in staff satisfaction related to support and education (Cook Gotay, 1984). The reader is advised to refer to this informative study for the detail it provides to assist with program planning and evaluation.

Issues in Palliative Care in Canada

1. Education for Palliative Care

The nurse's role in palliative care is central by virtue of its continuity and its intimacy (Hockey, 1978). It is a very personal care because often these patients need great assistance with activities such as eating, bathing and elimination. Since the incidence of terminal illness related to cancer increases with advancing age (Ajemian and Mount, 1981), nurses and physicians are caring not only for terminally ill patients but also the elderly. To give such personal care to an elderly patient or to any patient without damage to his/her dignity and self-respect demands a sound knowledge of behavioural sciences, strong ability in establishing human relationships and high competence in the art of nursing (Hockey, 1978). Students must be educated to value these aspects of nursing care regardless of the setting.

Physicians and nurses require professional education in the emotional and psychological implications of death. How do you teach nurses and physicians to give the emotional support that is required in palliative care? How do you teach, for example, nursing students to deal with their feelings about death as well as the feelings being expressed by their dying patients, whether these patients are in palliative care or intensive care units?

The United Kingdom has addressed the need for education in terminal care with the development of the English National Board course, Care of the Dying Patient and his Family. This is an eight-week course designed for nurses who have received their basic nursing education. Recently a further course has been developed which offers further education in this area at a more advanced level. In addition, facilities such as the Wade Study Centre at St Christopher's Hospice provide many educational opportunities for nurses, residents and other health care professionals involved in terminal care. Canada has recognized that many more physicians specifically trained in palliative care are needed to improve the quality of pain and other symptom control for patients. Similar to the United Kingdom, it is the general practitioner who is the physician caring for the terminal patient who remains at home. It is therefore essential that he/she understands the palliative care system and how to use it as well as the principles of palliative care.

Multidisciplinary team work is a strong component of hospice/ palliative care both in the United Kingdom and in Canada. The author's experience with hospice and continuing care nurses in the United Kingdom illustrated the importance of nurses working within a team where there is mutual respect for each other's roles and opinions. Implicit within team work is the assumption that each member asks for support when necessary and provides support to other team members as required. Education programs for health professionals need to emphasize the skills and attitudes required to work in a multidisciplinary team whether in palliative care or intensive care. The aim in many palliative care services in Canada is that of an interdisciplinary team where the person on the team best suited to help the patient progress does so. This might entail a physiotherapist teaching a volunteer the exercises the patient requires if the volunteer has the best rapport with the patient.

A task force report on palliative care in Ontario emphasized that physicians and nurses should be exposed to the principles and philosophies of palliative care as well as the fundamentals of pain management and other symptom control. This report also stressed the need to develop undergraduate and graduate teaching programs encompassing these concepts (Cousens, Andrewes and Dean, 1987). Some courses in Canada have been established to facilitate the education of health professionals in palliative care. The following are just isolated examples of programs offered. (1) an interdisciplinary certificate in palliative care is offered by Algonquin College in Ottawa. This is a post-secondary institution that offers full and part-time courses for many disciplines including nursing. (2) The University of Ottawa School of Nursing offers a nursing elective in palliative care. It is a three-credit course and is open to any third or fourth year nursing student as well as to registered nurses who are enrolled in the degree program. (3) The University of Manitoba in Winnipeg has fashioned the principles of palliative care into their generic nursing program under the umbrella of ameliorative nursing (University of Manitoba, 1984).

Some Canadian nurses have been able to take advantage of the educational links established with the United Kingdom, such as the intensive six-week hospice program whereby these nurses obtain both theory and clinical experience in British hospices.

Health and Welfare Canada has taken a step to educate the health professionals regarding the management of cancer pain, through a monograph published as a result of the expert advisory committee on the Management of Severe Chronic Pain in Cancer patients. The monograph discusses the reasons for poor pain control, such as lack of factual knowledge about analgesics. The differences between acute and chronic pain are highlighted as well as the principles of therapy in cancer pain. The steps of analgesia for mild to severe pain are clearly demonstrated as well as common therapeutic agents for cancer pain. The principles of narcotic administration in cancer patients are illustrated as are the myths about analgesia. The concept of total pain is made clear as is the need for a team approach for the management of total pain (*Cancer Pain*, 1984). This monograph also discusses the controversial subject of the use of diamorphine for cancer patients. Although readily available in the United Kingdom, Canada has introduced Diamorphine only recently in clinical trials with cancer patients. Although the debate about the use of this narcotic continues, health professionals are increasingly aware of the principles of pain management through educational efforts such as that produced by Health and Welfare Canada.

Integration of the philosophy and principles of palliative care into health science education will benefit patients and staff in providing health care that is sensitive and caring no matter what the setting.

2. The Setting for Palliative Care

It has been discussed thus far that hospice/palliative care can take many forms, including free-standing structures, palliative care units and palliative care services. In a country the size of Canada, the creation of multiple free-standing hospices would be an enormous undertaking financially as well as structurally. Two questions must be answered. First, is it more cost-effective to improve home care services and improve or develop services within hospitals rather than build separate hospices? Second, would patients and families choose the hospice option over the hospital if the choice were available (Cousens, Andrewes and Dean, 1987)? Further research which evaluates patient satisfaction with services and the cost-effectiveness of services is warranted and timely. As palliative care continues to expand in Canada, a choice must be made by the concerned individuals whether to develop a unit, a service or a free-standing structure. Each approach raises its own issues. If a unit is formed within a hospital, it tends to become a specialized area just as is an intensive care unit. This raises the question of whether palliative care is a specialty or a philosophy of care that should be applied to all patients. One of the advantages of a special unit is that staff are educated in the needs of the patients and family. A disadvantage is that the unit must be specifically built and staffed. A consideration in units *versus* services is that of the patient's choice in terms of which institution to be admitted to. For example, if patients are from a farming community, they may have gone to the local hospital for medical care most of their life. Patients may prefer the option of returning to their local hospital which has a palliative care service rather than be admitted to an entirely different facility that has a specific unit.

If a hospital has a palliative care service, all nurses on the ward where the terminal patient is located would learn, for example, about pain control through the team of the service. The patient in a palliative care service is not hospitalized just with patients who also have cancer, but rather is exposed to patients with a variety of problems. Both a service and a specific unit offer the advantage of fast access to human and technical resources when needed.

The disadvantages of a palliative care service can be that the philosophy of active treatment hospitals and that of palliative care are not in concert. It thus can become a challenge to prevent palliative care patients from being provided active treatment. The end result could be situations in which there is insufficient control over the environment and the decisions made by medical staff. In response to this latter concern, there is now a move in Canada for legislation of the 'Do not resuscitate' order. Specific palliative care units have policies for patient treatment. To protect patients who are being cared for in active treatment areas from interventions they would otherwise not choose to have, this order will be written by the physician. The nurse caring for the patient must discuss the order with the patient and family so that it is understood by all parties concerned.

Free-standing hospices are the other option. As in the United Kingdom, patients remain until death occurs or until they are able to return home again once pain and other problems are under control. They can also allow families an emotional and physical rest from care by admitting the patient for a short period. Beds are less costly as less expensive technology is involved (Cousens, Andrewes and Dean, 1987).

The cost of building large numbers of these structures in Canada has been discussed. Hospices, without public education, can generate the reaction that they are houses for the dying. There is also the concern of quality control with rapid proliferation of hospices. This debate can continue in the United Kingdom as well with the current structure of both free-standing hospices and continuing care units.

3. The Patients for Palliative Care

Historically, hospices have dealt with individuals suffering from conditions other than neoplastic disease. Our Lady's Hospice in Dublin, Ireland (1879) and St Joseph's Hospice in London (1905) accepted patients with long-term illness (Saunders, Walsh and Smith, 1981). This is also true of today's hospice. For example, when St Christopher's Hospice opened (1967), 10 per cent of its ward beds were allocated for patients with advanced neurological illnesses such as motor neurone disease (Saunders, Walsh and Smith, 1981). Does the acceptance of these patients move the hospice from its role as facility that provides terminal care to one that provides chronic care as well? The issue here becomes the definition of scope. What is meant by hospice/palliative care and at what stage in any fatal illness does a person become terminally ill? Blues and Zerwekh (1984) believe palliative care is that which provides the most current treatment to relieve the symptoms and distress of the disease process, whereas hospice care continues into bereavement. In Canada, hospice and palliative care are terms which are frequently used interchangeably for care of the terminally ill patient and family. Echlin (1982) believes terminal care is beyond palliative care and that nursing management must vary significantly between the two.

This issue will be discussed utilizing two groups of patients with non-malignant disease who are currently admitted into hospice/palliative care.

Patients with amyotrophic lateral sclerosis (motor neurone disease) are increasingly being cared for under palliative care in Canada. This disease is characterized by the progressive wasting of muscles, which can occur rapidly over months or extend for several years. Impairment of mobility, difficulty with speech and respiratory failure are the major physical problems (Zimmerman, 1986). The psychological needs that can be met by a palliative care approach include help with communication, help with family stress and role adjustment and the maintenance of some control over one's life (Kristjanson, Nelson and Henteleff, 1987). The question remains — at what stage in this person's illness should they be admitted to palliative care? If the disease is progressing slowly but respiratory difficulties develop then active treatment with mechanical ventilation may be carried out. If this ventilatory assistance is needed for some time it may be difficult for staff to care for this patient (Kristjanson, Nelson and Henteleff, 1987). Palliative care and the scope it wishes to take will have to address these problems.

The other group of patients that are being considered for palliative management are those with acquired immune deficiency syndrome. AIDS is increasingly a concern in Canada, with over 1000 patients having been diagnosed with the disease as of April 1987. There is varied opinion as to how active the treatment of these patients should be since the disease is fatal, with most people dying within one to two years of diagnosis. Initially many hospitals encouraged active treatment and the patient was admitted to the intensive care unit and often ventilated. Presently there appears to be a shift from intensive care to palliative care. Downing (1986) has raised important issues to consider if the shift to palliative management continues: (1) should hospice palliative care be provided at the time of diagnosis or later as the patient's condition worsens; (2) will acceptance of these patients alter the criteria for admission to this type of care; (3) can the peaceful atmosphere of hospice/palliative care be maintained while at the same time taking measures to minimize the fear of contagion to other patients and staff; (4) will support be available to handle the fears and possible biases of staff; (5) as the number of these patients increases, will separate facilities be built or additions made.

The United Kingdom is attempting to deal with some of these issues. Action is being taken to provide facilities for AIDS patients in the form of specialized units such as at Charing Cross Hospital in London. The development of free-standing structures is also being considered, such as the conversion of unused schools. The mandate of most hospices continues to be primarily for cancer patients in the United Kingdom.

In Canada, the eventual aim is to get the AIDS patient home. The crux lies in dealing with a patient population that is increasing and which may have little family support.

Again, the question remains as to whether patients who have conditions such as AIDS or motor neurone disease should be cared for in the same facilities as those with terminal cancer. The answer to this question will be a challenge to care-givers.

Nurses at the Forefront of Palliative Care

Nurses are pivotal in palliative care. It is nurses who frequently have stimulated the enthusiasm in communities to develop palliative care programs in regions across Canada. Nurses are increasingly the coordinators of the palliative care team. Canadian nursing associations are often the voice for concerned nurses who want palliative care a high priority in health care. For example, the Registered Nurses Association of Ontario has made the following resolutions regarding palliative care: (1) that nursing services be extended on a shift basis regardless of the ability to pay; (2) that the Registered Nurses Association lobby the government of Ontario to develop a plan and provide funding for the delivery of palliative care in Ontario; (3) that the Registered Nurses Association of Ontario consider as a priority for the 1987 budget year the development of a position paper on the role of the nurse in palliative care (*RNAO News*, 1986).

Nursing Models and Palliative Care

Conceptual models are used in nursing as general guides for the organization of nursing knowledge and for the design and implementation of clinical nursing practice, educational programs and research projects (Logan, 1986). Logan (1986) of the University of Ottawa School of Nursing has utilized the Roy model to determine if the model is appropriate for palliative care nursing and if it can be applied effectively to improve the care of the dying person and family. An assessment guide using the Roy model for the palliative care patient has been developed.

The Betty Neuman Systems model has been used in the Hospice of Windsor, Ontario. The hospice is a palliative care service within a hospital and there is strong community involvement. The model with its systems framework provides a sound approach for organizing effective inter- and multidisciplinary assessments and interventions for the palliative care patient and family (Echlin, 1982).

The Roy model has also been used for terminal care patients in the United Kingdom. Chadderton (1986) found it offered a conceptually compatible framework for use in the UK for terminally ill patients and their families.

Conclusion

The present is a very exciting time in terms of the development of palliative care in Canada. Great strides have been made in the development of services and many more will be provided. Much work has been done in the education of health professionals and research is continuing into the best methods for pain control as well as into patient, family and care provider satisfaction with services. The future holds much promise for nurses in the field of palliative care. Their role as coordinator of care provided in a team will also expand their role as patient advocate. The challenge is there for nursing to take.

Acknowledgements

The author would like to thank Professor Marion Logan of the University of Ottawa for her assistance with this chapter. The author would also like to extend her deep appreciation to the nursing sisters and staff of all the hospices and continuing care units visited in the United Kingdom. They so graciously opened their doors and their hearts to a Canadian.

References

Ajemian, I., and Mount, B.M. (1981) Hospice as a style for living. In Saunders, Dame C., Summers, D.H., and Teller, N. (eds) *Hospice: The Living Idea.* Edward Arnold, London, pp. 19–31.

Blues, A.G., and Zerwekh, J.V. (1984) *Hospice and Palliative Nursing Care.* Grune & Stratton, London.

Chadderton, H. (1986) A stress adaptation model in terminal care. In Kershaw, B., and Salvage, J. (eds) *Models for Nursing.* Wiley, London, pp. 69–79.

Cook Gotay, C. (1984) *Calgary's Home Care Program: A Descriptive Study of the Third Year.* University of Calgary, Calgary.

Cousens, D., Andrewes, P., and Dean, G. (1987). Palliative care: Developing a comprehensive system in Ontario. A discussion paper, *Journal of Palliative Care*, 2 (2), 44–51.

Dionne, L., and staff members (1986) La Maison Michel Sarrazin, *The American Journal of Hospice Care*, 3 (3), 27–32.

Downing, G.M. (1986) Palliative AIDS care — To be or not to be, *Journal of Palliative Care*, 1 (2), 32–40.

Echlin, D.J. (1982) Palliative care and the Neuman model. In Neuman, B. (ed.) *The Neuman Systems Model.* Appleton Century Crofts, Conn., pp. 257–259.

Doyle, D., (ed.) *Terminal Care.* Churchill Livingstone, Edinburgh, pp. 42–51.

Kristjanson, L.J., Nelson, F., and Henteleff, P. (1987) Palliative care for individuals with amyotrophic lateral sclerosis, *Journal of Palliative Care*, 2 (2), 28–34.

Logan, M. (1986) Palliative care nursing: Applicability of the Roy model, *Journal of Palliative Care*, 1 (2), 18–24.

Manning, M. (1984) *The Hospice Alternative*. Souvenir Press, London.

Parkes, C.M. (1985) Terminal care: Home, hospital, or hospice? *Lancet*, Jan. 19, 155–157.

Saunders, Dame C., Walsh, T.D., and Smith, M. (1981) Hospice care in motor neuron disease. In Saunders, Dame C., Summers, D.H., and Teller, N. (eds) *Hospice: The Living Idea*. Edward Arnold, London, pp. 126–147.

Scott, J. (1981) Canada: Hospice care in Canada. In Saunders, Dame C., Summers, D.H., and Teller, N. (eds) *Hospice: The Living Idea*. Edward Arnold, London, pp. 176–180.

Stephenson-Cino, P.M., Roe, D.J., Latimer, E., Walton, L., and Thomson, J.N. (1987) An examination of palliative shift care funding, *Journal of Palliative Care*, **2** (2), 13–17.

Zimmerman, J.M. (1986) *Hospice: Complete Care for the Terminally Ill*, 2nd edn. Urban & Schwarzenberg, Maryland.

Reports

Cancer Pain (1984) A Report of the Expert Advisory Committee on the Management of Severe Chronic Pain in Cancer Patients. Health and Welfare Canada.

Ottawa–Carleton Regional Palliative Care Association (1986) Ottawa, Ontario.

RNAO News (October 1986) Registered Nurses Association of Ontario, Toronto.

University of Manitoba School of Nursing Calendar (1984).

Part 3   Psychological Care

Nursing Issues and Research in Terminal Care
Edited by J. Wilson-Barnett and J. Raiman
© 1988 John Wiley & Sons Ltd.

CHAPTER 3

Bereavement Care

JUDITH HILL

Introduction

Grief is a recognized pattern of emotional reaction following bereavement, the loss of a loved person. Most people will cope with their grief through the help of supportive families, friends and social groups such as churches. However, changes in society such as rising divorce rates, increased numbers of working mothers and greater mobility which separates generations geographically and fragments family groups have decreased the amount of support available and other ways are having to be found to help the bereaved (Parkes, 1986).

Professionals from a variety of disciplines are becoming involved in supporting the bereaved. Nurses in hospice care, the community, and hospital are developing skills in this area, drawing on research material gathered by other disciplines. This chapter will review the work of a number of experts in the field, identifying the nature of grief, its effects, the process of mourning, and ways of facilitating grief, before going on to explore the nurse's role in helping the bereaved in hospital and at home and the work of specialist nurses, nursing education in bereavement, the bereaved nurse and areas for nursing research.

The Nature of Grief

Grief is the reaction to loss (Parkes, 1986). In order to understand the nature of grief, the way in which people first become attached needs to be understood. There is a mystery in the close bonds which exist beween people (Heike, 1985). Attachment theory (Bowlby, 1979) offers a way of looking at the making of strong affectional bonds with others and helps the understanding of the strong emotional reaction which follows when those bonds are threatened or broken (Worden, 1983). The attachments arise from a need for safety and security, developing early in life and directed towards a small number of individuals. Acute anxiety and strong protest follow the disappearance of the attachment figure (Worden, 1983). The patterns of attachment give meaning to life. If they are disrupted by change and loss the individual is unable to experience life as meaningful and is plunged into grief (Marris, 1986).

Grief is a natural process, the price paid for love (Freud, 1917; Parkes, 1986). It has been variably described as the response to the loss of meaning (Marris, 1986); a physical injury or blow (Parkes, 1986); a psychological wound or departure from the state of health and well-being (Engel, 1961). Many authors agree that it is a process that requires time for healing or recovery to take place (e.g. Parkes, 1986; Engel, 1962; Marris, 1986).

The Effects of Grief

Grief has effects on an individual physically, emotionally, spiritually, and socially. There is evidence that the bereaved, especially widowers, are at greater risk of dying during the first year of bereavement than the normal population of comparable age. Young, Benjamin and Wallis (1963) found a peak of mortality in widowers 54 years old and upwards during the first year of bereavement. After looking at six major studies, Osterweiss et al. (1984) found men up to the age of 75 were at greater risk of death than their married counterparts. There was a significant rise in the death rate among widows in the first three months and widowers in the first twelve months following the death of their spouse in a study by Mellstrom et al. (1982). Parents and grandparents have also been found to be at risk when a child has died (Rees and Lutkins, 1967; Roskin, 1984). The most frequent cause of death is heart disease (Parkes, 1986). Other causes of raised mortality rates in the bereaved are cirrhosis of the liver, infectious diseases, accidents and suicides (Helsing et al., 1981).

Loss has been cited as the cause of much physical and mental illness because these have occurred shortly after the event. Marris (1958) and Hobson (1964) reported the general health of widows had deteriorated with a large number of symptoms listed, including headaches, digestive disorders, rheumatism and asthma. Hinton (1972) gives a similar lengthy list of physical symptoms: fatigue, insomnia, loss of appetite, loss of weight, headache, breathlessness, palpitations, blurred vision. Lindemann (1944) was the first to describe the symptomatology of acute grief, and 25 years later Parkes (1970) found a 63 per cent rise in visits to the GP by younger widows with complaints of insomnia, depression or anxiety. These physical symptoms reflect the responses of the body to the psychological stress of bereavement — Parkes (1986) likens the response to the alarm reaction which prepares the individual for flight or fight. The emotional component of the response includes feelings of fear (Lewis, 1961), disbelief, anxiety, pining, waves of yearning (Parkes, 1986), misery and despair, loss of concentration, self-doubt, guilt, shame, anger, wanting to blame someone, even a feeling of relief (Hinton, 1972). In a personal account of bereavement, Heike (1985) describes an inner chaos, with swings of mood, pangs and yearning, apathy and detachment. The present seems meaningless, the future pointless and threatening. Certain societies provide the bereaved with ways of dealing with their grief and maintaining status (Neuberger, 1987). The western industrial society often adds to the person's sense of loss by stigmatizing the single person; many widows' lives are so bound up with their husbands that they lose status and role on his death. As a single person Heike (1985) felt her grief at the death of her flatmate was misunderstood; people felt it was out of proportion. Other social implications of grief include financial loss or gain, loss of patterns of behaviour and the need to take on a new identity and learn new skills.

Abnormal Grief Reactions

There is a fine balance between normal and abnormal grief reactions. Pathology is related more to the depth or length of the reaction rather than to any particular behaviour (Worden, 1983). The reaction may become prolonged, with the person stuck, perhaps unable to let go of anger at the circumstances of the death. The reaction may be delayed and then precipitated by another crisis or loss, when it may appear disproportionate to the nature of the secondary loss (Parkes, 1980). Exaggerated reactions can occur when the normal response takes on a neurotic form of emotional distress, such as phobias about being left alone or in an enclosed space, phobias about dirt, death or dying (Hinton, 1972; Worden, 1983). Quoting Lazare (1979), Worden (1983) lists twelve clues to detecting an abnormal grief reaction. No one clue is conclusive, but a combination of several can point to the diagnosis. The list includes such signs as an unwillingness to move the possessions of the deceased after a suitable time lapse; physical symptoms similar to the condition from which the deceased suffered; unaccountable sadness at a certain time each year; avoidance of death-related activities or rituals at the time of the death (Worden, 1983). Further abnormal features would be a tendency to idealize the dead person to the point of idolization and the preserving of possessions and customs, even making a shrine of his room or house. Queen Victoria showed such behaviour on the death of Prince Albert (Gorer, 1965).

Coping with Grief: The Process of Mourning

The process of grief constitutes a series of adjustments which a number of authors have tried to organize into stages, phases or tasks. Engel (1962) describes three stages:

1. Shock and disbelief
2. Developing awareness
3. Restitution

Parkes (1972) delineates four phases:

1. Numbness
2. Pining
3. Depression
4. Recovery

Worden (1983) proposes four tasks of mourning.

1. Acceptance of the reality of the loss
2. Experience of the pain of grief
3. Adjustment to an environment without the deceased
4. Withdrawal of emotional energy and reinvestment in another relationship

There is considerable similarity of thought between the schemes. Worden (1983) prefers the term 'task' to 'phase' as it implies the bereaved can take an active part in their recovery and this view is supported by Parkes (1986) as he puts forward the components of grief work.

Marris (1986) sees two fundamental impulses at work in grief:

1. To return to the time before death
2. To reach forward to a state of mind where the past is forgotten

There is a tension between these impulses; first one wins then the other. By moving forward in jerky steps the bereaved are able to let go of the person but retain for the future the values they represented in their relationships. All this takes time, usually one to two years, sometimes longer (Engel, 1962; Parkes, 1972). It is recognized that mourning is completed when the positive and negative aspects of the relationship can be recalled realistically and without pain (Worden, 1983; Engel, 1962).

The Determinants of Grief

Having looked at the range of effects in grief and the process of mourning, the question needs to be asked: is it possible to predict how a particular individual will react? Are there certain factors which will give an indication who is likely to have a severe reaction in bereavement? The evidence points to a number of indicators which can be used to predict the course of grief. Worden (1983) gives a taxonomy for determining grief patterns.

1. Who the person was
2. The nature of the attachment
   (a) Its strength
   (b) Its security
   (c) The presence of any ambivalence in the relationship
3. The mode of death
   — accidental, natural, suicidal, homicidal
   — near or at a distance
   — sudden or anticipated
4. Historical antecedents
   — previous grief reaction
   — history of depressive illness
5. Personality variables
   — age/sex
   — types of coping strategies in anxiety/stress
6. Social variables
   — ethnic and/or religious background
   — secondary gain to the bereaved

Marris (1986) suggests four conditions before, at, or after the loss that can be expected to influence a person's ability to reconstitute meaning, namely, the childhood experience of attachment, doubtful or unresolved meaning of the loss, an opportunity to prepare for or predict the loss, supportive or stressful events after the loss. Younger and middle-aged women are expected to have severe reactions and the loss of a child as discussed in another paper can present great difficulties (Hinton, 1972). Thus recovery from bereavement varies with the circumstance of the loss, the nature of the loss and the past history of the bereaved. In assessing how an individual will do, Marris poses several questions.

1. How can the person make sense of the loss?
2. Is the loss intelligible, i.e. consistent with a worthwhile world?
3. Can any purpose be derived from it?
4. How conflicted or ambiguous was the meaning of what was lost?
5. What interpretation of loss is the underlying structure of meaning likely to support?
6. How do present relationships, or their lack, help or hinder the task of working all this out?

Marris (1986) contends that the intensity of the involvement rather than love governs the intensity of grief. Thus the widow of a man who worked on an oil-rig, however much she may have loved her husband, is likely to adapt to his death more quickly and with less disruption to her life than the woman who was wife and business partner to a newsagent, working and living with him 24 hours a day, so that his death means that everything in her life will be different.

Our society places a particular emphasis on different relationships so that the following could represent a declining order of severity of bereavement: the death of a spouse, child, parent, sibling or friend. However, there is a need not to make assumptions from such a list, as a person's grief may be deepened by misunderstanding the nature of a relationship; for example, Heike (1985) found that she was getting messages both implicitly and explicitly that grief for a friend should be less profound than that for a relative.

Facilitating Grief

It is not up to us to say whether someone's grief is or is not legitimate. Grief is grief and needs a healer (Heike, 1985). How is the healer to function? Speck (1985) supports the view that people need to grieve in their own way. Those who want to help need to build a relationship which takes into account the bereaved person's culture, expectations and the value they place on the lost relationship, and offer them a safe place to express their thoughts and feelings.

Worden (1983) lists some principles to apply in facilitating grief:

1. Let the person talk to help them realize the loss.
2. Allow the expression of strong feelings — anger, guilt, anxiety, sadness, helplessness.
3. Help the person to cope with living on their own.
4. Help the person to let go emotionally of the deceased.
5. Allow time for grief. Contact the person at critical times, e.g. three months, twelve months, etc.
6. Reassure them that their behaviour is normal.
7. Treat them as an individual.
8. Provide support over time, refer on to relevant support group.
9. Watch for maladaptive reactions such as the use of drugs or alcohol.
10. Refer for more specialized help if abnormal reactions begin to occur.

The general consensus is that medication ought to be used sparingly to relieve anxiety or insomnia rather than to mask a normal distress. Funerals can help facilitate grief (Speck, 1985), as they draw to the bereaved other people who acknowledge the death and allow the bereaved to realize their new status. The funeral can reflect the meaning of the life of the deceased (Worden, 1983).

Parkes (1980) describes a number of ways to organize the support of the bereaved: firstly through professional services by doctors, nurses, psychologists, or social workers for individuals or groups; secondly through trained volunteers, supported by professionals; thirdly through self-help groups, where those who suffered a similar bereavement reach out to the newly bereaved, e.g. the Compassionate Friends, Cruse, National Association of Widows. Many hospice services use a combination of all three.

The Nurse's Role in Bereavement

Having looked at an overview of what is known about grief and bereavement, the need is to look more specifically at the literature and research which refers to the nurse's role in bereavement care. There is little actual nursing research on the topic, although reference is made in a number of nursing books on care of the dying to the needs of families and the process of grief (Charles-Edwards, 1983; Robbins, 1983; Copperman, 1983). These give guidelines on common hospice practice in preparing the families of the terminally ill and ways of helping them begin anticipatory grief work. There is some research in terminal care which examines bereavement care and how nurses feel about supporting families of the dying.

The nurse needs to know the way people react in the early stages of grief and also later in bereavement as she will come into contact with the bereaved in a variety of situations. In hospital, she may be the one to break the news of the death or will support families as they keep vigil by those known to be dying. She is responsible for initiating the formalities of collecting property and the death certificate. The nurse can meet the bereaved in midwifery, accident and emergency departments, intensive care units, the paediatric, geriatric and psychiatric wards, as well as in general medicine and surgical units. As the research discussed earlier has shown, many bereaved people become seriously ill with heart or other disorders, and so many of the patients in hospital will be people in the throes of grief, whose reaction to their present illness may be exaggerated by their grief reaction.

Likewise in the community, the district nurse will continue to support the families of her patients who have died. The health visitor may be called upon to support parents following a stillbirth or the accidental death of a child, or it may be that the mothers of healthy children whom she is visiting will have experienced the death of a parent or husband and will look to her for help. The health visitor will also be involved where the parent of young children has died.

Care of the Bereaved in Hospital

Other chapters have considered the care of families in terminal illness and highlighted the need for good communication by staff with the families and to take the opportunity to help families begin to mourn. Involving families in the care can be a help later in bereavement (Hampe, 1975; Richmond and Waisman, 1955). This chapter will look more at the nurse's role at and after death.

Following death there is a procedure for the practical tasks of care of the body and the collection of the patient's property, and the signing of the death certificate. Alongside these activities there is the informing and support of the relatives. If they were not present at the death the nurse may have to make arrangements for them to view the body, which often entails a complicated procedure with porters and mortuary attendants. From the reactions discussed earlier, what the bereaved need is time to take in the reality of the death and to say goodbye to their loved one. They are often numb and bewildered, and the hurry of acute wards, the hastily given instructions on how to collect property and the death certificate, only adds to their bewilderment. Nurses may rush such procedures because they are afraid of their own emotions and find it difficult to support the bereaved (Hockley, 1983; Lewars, 1983). On the other hand, some nurses would like to do more, being concerned for relatives going home on their own. Some contact community liaison staff and ask them to inform the GP and/or health visitor. Some write to relatives or invite them for a follow-up discussion, e.g. Queen Alexandra Hospital, Portsmouth. Some hospitals give a copy of the DHSS leaflet *What To Do After a Death* and others have produced their own guidelines, including information on normal reactions in grief (McGuiness, 1986; Southampton General Hospital) which they hand to the bereaved to take home and read at their leisure.

Despite these efforts, there has been much criticism of the care of bereaved relatives in hospital, especially when the death has been sudden. The Health Service Ombudsman has regularly received complaints which he has been forced to uphold. They often relate to poor communication by medical and nursing staff, or are to do with the administrative procedures for collection of property and the death certificate.

Robertson (1978) commented in the report of her study tour that relatives she spoke to felt they had not been allowed to remain at the bedside as long as they would have wished. They also resented the clothes being put in the ubiquitous polythene bag, still around in 1987. Many expressed a preference to collect the property from the ward where the nurses were familiar rather than from a stranger in a strange office. She explained the part played by the general atmosphere of the hospital. A welcoming and interested reception at the entrance could do much to relieve the anxiety of frightened relatives in what to many is an alien environment. Hockley (1983), having found little research available on the care of relatives, included them in her study to evaluate the care of the dying on general hospital wards. She found many were exhausted by caring for a terminally ill patient at home. A large group had had little or no discussion with the doctors and lacked information about what was happening. Nearly all the wards studied had no private room for seeing relatives. All these factors were inhibiting anticipatory mourning.

Lunt's (1985) work comparing hospital and hospices reported that spouse stress and anxiety were relieved in the hospice but were increased in the hospital. This seemed to reflect the fact that in hospital the nurses and doctors had different goals for the patient and were giving conflicting information to the relatives. He also found the relatives of hospital patients were more anxious and felt unsupported at the time of death, and in fact were less likely to be present at the death, than the relatives of hospice patients. There was no difference between the two groups in the grief reaction at six months. It requires more research to see if there is a difference later on in bereavement.

Various ways of tackling some of these problems are being tried. Lewisham Hospital set up a volunteer scheme where the volunteer acted like a supportive relative, accompanying the isolated bereaved home, making a cup of tea and providing a listening ear (Keyte, Meade and Nye, 1980). Guidelines related to care of the dying have been published by the King's Fund (Henley, 1986) which include advice to health authorities on the care of relatives at and after death and a similar document has been produced by the National Association of Health Authorities (NAHA, 1987). Following the DHSS circular HC/ 4/87 requesting all health authorities to formulate plans for care of the dying and their families, it is hoped some of the ideas suggested in these two documents, such as better communication with relatives and smoother, speedier administrative procedures, will be put into practice and there will be an improvement in hospital care of the bereaved.

McGuiness (1986), a nurse/bereavement counsellor, made a study in a previous post in an accident and emergency unit to elicit to what extent needs of the bereaved determined their care. She found little evidence that a person's cultural background was taken into account in nursing practice, so that some rituals practised by members of the multiracial community in relation to the dead were in danger of being violated. She found doctors spent three minutes with the relatives after telling the news of a death and the nurse averaged ten minutes with the bereaved before they left the unit. The nurse actively discouraged the families from viewing the body. There was little privacy for the grieving relatives in the open-plan unit. None of the staff had received training in how to break bad news and they found overt emotional reactions difficult to deal with, even though a large proportion of the staff recognized the need to facilitate expressions of grief.

In her current post as a bereavement counsellor McGuiness often acts as a liaison nurse between the relatives and the resuscitation staff, keeping them informed of what is happening and preparing them for a poor outcome. Having built a relationship with the family she is usually the one to break the news of the death, with a doctor coming in later to answer questions. She stays with the family until they are ready to leave, linking with chaplain, social worker or other relatives as necessary. She informs the GP and offers to ring the family the next day. This seems to be a good model for other units to follow. Such roles need to be evaluated to see their effectiveness.

A number of hospitals have set up hospital support teams for the care of the terminally ill (Bates *et al.*, 1981) which, following hospice philosophy, take relatives as part of their responsibility and set up bereavement support groups, as well as being available to relatives before and after death. Some of these teams have been evaluated in the study by Lunt and Yardley (1987).

Care of the Bereaved in the Community

The district nurse, caring for a terminally ill patient at home, often feels a responsibility to go on visiting the family once the patient has died. Copperman (1983) recommends a visit on the day following the death to collect equipment and express sympathy. Some nurses will attend the funeral and then continue to visit according to the needs they perceive in the family (Reid, 1982). Visits at one month, three months and on the anniversary of the death are recommended (Copperman, 1983). Others visit randomly but with some emphasis around the anniversary (Robertson, 1978).

The follow-up of sudden deaths in hospital of people unknown to the community services seems to rely on a referral from the GP; however, this may not be forthcoming until a crisis arises (Robertson, 1978).

Some people feel nurses are not comfortable with the non-practical role which bereavement support requires and so may not be the most suitable people to be involved. Although the health visitors have usually made the adjustment from 'doing' to 'being around', their caseloads often preclude them being heavily involved in bereavement care. The development of Macmillan nursing services and home care support teams for the terminally ill in the last decade offered a way out of this problem, but as the next section shows they too have limitations.

The Role of Specialist Nurses in Bereavement

In this country there has been little evaluation of the role of specialist nurses in caring for the bereaved. A study of home care services (Ward,

1985) excluded bereavement care, although acknowledging that it was an area of the work of such services. Sims (unpublished) included comments on bereavement visiting by the terminal care nurses she interviewed. Most referred to the fact that bereavement support for families of past patients had to take a lower priority to providing support to current patients and their families. Some mentioned bereavement evenings and a befriending service run by volunteers.

A large, detailed survey of home care teams and hospital support teams (Lunt and Yardley, 1987) sheds more light on the subject. Most nurses interviewed aimed to visit at least once or twice after the patient had died, and then assessed the relatives' need and would continue visiting or refer on to a professional or voluntary agency. Thirty-four per cent of the services studied provided bereavement evenings and some used or were planning to use volunteers for a bereavement service.

Bereavement follow-up was an objective for nearly all the services, but was generally only partly achieved for similar reasons to Sims' study. Many of the nurses were dissatisfied with the bereavement follow-up and there was a lot of variation both within and between teams in the time given to this area of work. Interestingly, bereavement was seen as a source of stress to the nurses in two ways. Firstly, they themselves felt bereaved at the loss of patients, especially when several died in a short period of time; and secondly, the relatives' grief distressed them. Such comments may reflect a lack of training in this area of care (see below). There is still much unknown about the effects of working with the dying and bereaved on these nurses and how they should be involved in bereavement care.

Nurse Education in Bereavement Care

Dealing with death and dying is becoming an accepted part of the nursing curriculum. Lewars (1983) introduced a varied programme of videos, discussions and ward teaching on the subject of death and dying. However, there is no evidence that dealing with relatives before, at or after death formed part of the programme, despite the learners rating talking with relatives as the fourth most stressful aspect of care.

Field and Kitson (1986) surveyed schools of nursing to see how well nurses are being prepared to deal with death, dying patients and bereaved relatives. They found a range of time on RGN courses from two to 42 hours, with a mean of ten hours. A range of teaching methods were used and over 90 per cent of RGN, EN and degree courses included bereavement as one of the topics taught. The schools felt the teaching given had helped to reduce learner anxiety but Field and Kitson were sceptical as to the application in the wards because of the pressure of work.

Hockley (1983) found nurses were coping well with the physical care of the terminally ill patients, but care of their families presented difficulties, supporting findings in other studies by Whitfield (1979) and Birch (1979). The learners in Hockley's study would have liked more ward-based teaching.

Sims (unpublished) interviewed specialist terminal care nurses who had undertaken the then Joint Board of Clinical Nursing Studies course 930 Care of the dying patient and his family, to see how useful they had found it as training for their work and to identify any limitations. Surprisingly, despite an objective on bereavement, several nurses in this pilot study mentioned there had been little teaching on family or bereavement care and identified the fact that they would be pursuing a course in bereavement in the near future. The present English National Board course 931 still has an objective on bereavement and the new 285 Specialist course lists in the content to be covered normal and abnormal grief reactions and the setting up of a bereavement service. These newer courses need to be evaluated to see whether specialist nurses are now feeling more prepared to be involved in bereavement care as a result of the courses designed to meet their needs.

The Bereaved Nurse

The nurse herself, or her colleagues, will at some time face a bereavement in the family. Being aware of the likely reactions and what helps or hinders the grief process will help her to deal with her own grief, or that of her colleagues. She may experience some difficulty, as the Royal College of Nursing Counselling Service has found (Crawley, 1984). The nurse is often the only health care professional in the family and is seen, or sees herself, as the one to shoulder much of the responsibility in relating to hospital or medical staff. She acts as the supporter and comforter of the rest of the family. Her grieving is often delayed, because she is expected to deal with the practicalities of death as she is used to dealing with such things. She may have to listen to anger against health professionals and become the scapegoat for the family's guilt.

The nurse is always on duty — at work and at home, supporting the family in its despair. Only as the family reaches some point of resolution and no longer needs the support does the nurse's own reaction to the loss begin to emerge. Crawley has identified that because of the time delay the reaction is often transferred, or seen as related to a different event. The nurse feels she is going mad and needs to have the situation explored and explained as a normal reaction, and the results of her delaying her own grieving, in order to care for and support her family. Crawley recommends counselling to be available for staff through the health authorities and more awareness of the needs of bereaved staff to be developed. Identifying the effects of bereavement on the nurse at work and the kind of support that her employers can offer would be an area for research.

Future Nursing Research in Bereavement Care

Some areas of difficulty for nurses in bereavement care have been identified in the literature, and further research is required to see how general these problems are and what strategies are the most effective for dealing with them. Suggested avenues for research are:

1. Nursing education programmes. Teaching content and methods in the basic curriculum require systematic evaluation as to their effectiveness in preparing nurse learners for dealing with bereaved families. The ward climate for learning this aspect of care also requires examination to see if what has been taught is being helped or hindered in clinical areas. Postbasic programmes, especially those on the care of the dying and their families, plus staff development courses on counselling similarly require good evaluation.
2. Ways of facilitating anticipatory mourning for relatives by nursing staff need to be identified and evaluated.
3. Ways of predicting where nurse involvement in bereavement care could be most effective need to be identified.
4. Specialist nurse roles in terminal care and bereavement counselling require systematic evaluation as to their effects on outcomes in bereavement.
5. The effects of bereavement on the nurse herself and her ability to fulfil her work role need to be identified. The place of compassionate leave, management and other support systems for the nurse could be evaluated.

References

Bates, T., Clarke, D.G., Hoy, A.M., and Laird, P.P. (1981) A new concept of hospice care. St Thomas's Terminal Care Support Team, *Lancet*, May 30, 1201–1203.

Birch, J. (1979) The anxious learners, *Nursing Mirror*, **148**, 17–22.

Bowlby, J. (1979) *The Making and Breaking of Affectional Bonds*. Tavistock, London.

Charles-Edwards, A. (1983) *Nursing Care of the Dying Patient*. Beaconsfield Publishers, Beaconsfield, Bucks.

Copperman, H. (1983) *Dying at Home*. Wiley, Chichester.

Crawley, P. (1984) Coping with the death of a close relative, *Nursing Standard*, October 25.

DHSS (1979) *What to Do After a Death*, DHSS Leaflet D.49.

Engel, G. L. (1961) Is grief a disease: A challenge for medical research, *Psychosomatic Medicine*, **23**, 18–22.

Engel, G.L. (1962) *Psychological Development in Health and Disease*. W.B. Saunders, Philadelphia.

Field, D., and Kitson, C. (1986) The practical reality, *Nursing Times*, March 19, 33–34.

Freud, S. (1917) *Mourning and Melancholia*. Standard edition, vol. 14.

Gorer, G. (1965) *Death, Grief and Mourning in Contemporary Britain*. Cresset, London.

Hampe, S.O. (1975) Needs of the grieving spouse in a hospital setting, *Nursing Research*, **24** (2), 113–119.

Heike, E. (1985) *A Question of Grief*. Hodder Christian Paperbacks, London.

Helsing, K.J. Saklo, M., and Comstock, G.W. (1981) Factors associated with mortality after widowhood, *American Journal of Public Health*, **71**, 802–809.

Henley, A. (1986) *Good Practice in Hospital Care for the Dying*, King's Fund Project Paper No. 61. King's Fund Publishing Office, London.

Hinton, J. (1972) *Dying*. Penguin, Harmondsworth.

Hobson, C.J. (1964) Widows of Blackton, *New Society*, 24 September, 13.

Hockley, J. (1983) *An Investigation to Identify Symptoms of Distress in the Terminally-Ill Patient and his/her Family in the General Medical Ward*. Nursing Research Papers No. 2, City and Hackney Health District, London.

Keyte, J., Meade, B., and Nye, (1980) Lewisham Bereavement Project. Death and the life that's left, *Health and Social Service Journal*, October 10, 1316–1318.

Lazare, A. (1979) Unresolved grief. In Lazare, A. (ed.) *Outpatient Psychiatry. Diagnosis and Treatment*. Williams & Wilkins, Baltimore.

Lewars, M. (1983) Caring for dying patients, *Nursing Mirror*, Oct. 5, 42–44.

Lewis, C.S. (1961) *A Grief Observed*. Faber & Faber, London.

Lindemann, E. (1944) Symptomatology and management of acute grief. *American Journal of Psychiatry*, **101**, 141.

Lunt, B. (1985) A Comparison of Hospice and Hospital Care for Terminally-Ill Cancer Patients and their Families. Unpublished research report.

Lunt, B., and Yardley, J. (1987) A Survey of Home Care Teams and Hospital

Support Teams for the Terminally ill. Unpublished report. Cancer Relief, Macmillan Fund, London.

Marris, P. (1958) *Widows and their Families*, Routledge & Kegan Paul, London.

McGuinness, S. (1986) Coping with death, *Nursing Times*, March 19, 29–31.

Mellstrom, D., Nilsson, A., Oden, A., Rundgren, Å, and Svanborg, A. (1982) Mortality among the widowed in Sweden, *Scandinavian Journal of Social Medicine*, **10**, 33–41.

NAHA (1987) *Care of the Dying*. National Association of Health Authorities, Birmingham.

Neuberger, J. (1987) *Caring for Dying People of Different Faiths*. Lisa Sainsbury Foundation Series, Austen Cornish Publishers, London.

Osterweiss, M., Solomon, F., and Green, M. (eds.) (1984) *Bereavement — Reactions, Consequences and Care*. National Academy Press, Washington DC.

Parkes, C.M. (1970) The first year of bereavement. A longitudinal study of the reaction of London widows to the death of their husband, *Psychiatry*, **33**, 444.

Parkes, C.M. (1972) *Bereavement. Studies of Grief in Adult Life*. Penguin, Harmondsworth.

Parkes, C.M. (1980) Bereavement counselling. Does it work, *British Medical Journal*, **281**, 3–6.

Parkes, C.M. (1986) *Studies of Grief in Adult Life*, 2nd edn. Penguin, Harmondsworth.

Rees, W.D., and Lutkins, S.G. (1967) Mortality of bereavement, *British Medical Journal*, **4**, 13.

Reid, G. (1982) District dialogue — bereavement, *Journal of District Nursing*, October 6.

Richmond, J.B., and Waisman, H.A. (1955) Psychologic aspects of management of children with malignant diseases, *American Journal of Disease in Childhood*, **89**, 42–47.

Robbins, J. (ed.) (1983) *Caring for the Dying Patient and the Family*. Harper & Row, London.

Robertson, A.E. (1978) *A Problem of Our Time*. Unpublished report of Primary Health Care Award, Smith & Nephew and Royal College of Nursing.

Roskin, M. (1984) A look at bereaved parents, *Bereavement Care*, **3**, 26–28.

Sims, M. (undated) *Nurse Training for Terminal Care*. Unpublished Report. Institute for Social Studies in Medical Care, London.

Speck, P. (1985) Religious and cultural aspects of dying, *Bereavement Care*, **4**, 28–30.

Ward, A.W.M. (1985) *Home Care Services for the Terminally-Ill*. A Report for the Nuffield Foundation, University of Sheffield.

Whitfield, S.A. (1979) A descriptive study of student nurses' ward experience with dying patients and their attitudes towards them. Manchester University thesis, Steinberg Collection Royal College of Nursing, London.

Worden, J.W. (1983) *Grief Counselling and Grief Therapy*. Tavistock, London.

Young, M., Benjamin, B., and Wallis, C. (1963) Mortality of widowers, *Lancet*, **2**, 454.

Nursing Issues and Research in Terminal Care
Edited by J. Wilson-Barnett and J. Raiman
© 1988 John Wiley & Sons Ltd.

CHAPTER 4

Dying Children and their Families

ALISON WHILE

Introduction

The death of a child in present times is an unusual event and inevitably evokes strong emotions. Childhood is perceived as a period of starting out in life and is rarely associated with serious ill-health and subsequent death. This chapter will review the available literature under the following headings: The problem; The needs of parents and children following diagnosis; The needs of the child during the illness; The needs of the family during the illness; The final illness; Bereavement.

The Problem

Childhood death is a relatively infrequent occurrence compared with its incidence earlier this century. Indeed, social development and advances in medical knowledge have eliminated many of the causes of death of yesteryear. Today the most vulnerable period of childhood is infancy, when disorders associated with prematurity and the birth process figure prominently together with sudden infant death syndrome. Deaths caused by accidents are another important feature of childhood mortality statistics (OPCS, 1982); however, such children die suddenly or after a very short illness and will therefore not be considered in this chapter.

Despite the relative infrequency of fatal disease in childhood, certain disorders are associated with a reduced life expectancy. Among childhood malignancies, tumours of the brain are the most numerous, followed by abdominal tumours and leukaemias (Dodge, 1974). Advances in medical care have greatly improved the survival rate of treated children (Hammond, 1986) although premature death due to malignancies continues. However, not all fatal illnesses of childhood are due to malignant disease and certain inherited disorders are responsible for a significant number of deaths in childhood. Examples of such diseases are Tay-Sachs disease, which is a degenerative disorder of the brain (Cowie, 1983), the X chromosome-linked disease of Duchenne muscular dystrophy (Dubowitz, 1978) and the recessively inherited condition of cystic fibrosis (Mearns, 1985). Although advances in therapy have helped children with cystic fibrosis to live longer so that an increasing number are reaching adult life, a large proportion continue to die in childhood from intractable respiratory disease. Congenital malformations also cause death in childhood, the most important of which is spina bifida. Further, some types of congenital heart disease are still not susceptible to successful treatment despite the progress which has been made in this field. Another cause of death in childhood is chronic renal failure, which may be the result of either congenital malformation or infective damage. Therapeutic measures and successful kidney transplantation have greatly reduced the mortality from this cause in recent years.

The Needs of Parents and Children following Diagnosis

The Parents

It would be naive to assume that the diagnosis of a life-threatening illness in a child might have anything but a traumatic effect upon parents. Such a diagnosis inevitably implies the loss of a normal, satisfying life full of joyful moments and, instead, hopelessness and pain. Barbor (1983) has argued that the diagnosis may not necessarily be a medical emergency but it is always an emotional emergency. Learning of the diagnosis is the first serious confrontation with the potential death of their child. Initial parental reactions to the diagnosis are very similar to the emotional and behavioural effects of normal grief subsequent to the loss of a loved one; however, the way in which parents respond varies widely and depends upon a large number of background factors including family background, available support and psychodynamic factors (Burton, 1974). The attribution of parental guilt is a particularly important consideration when the disease is an inherited disorder and the existence of a life-threatening congenital malformation confronts parents with the failure of their reproductive process. The management of this is discussed by Taylor (1982).

Myers (1983) has argued that the successful outcome of an informing interview depends upon the characteristics of the informer and the circumstances of the interview. He has suggested that one can learn to conduct an interview conveying 'bad news' with skill and sensitivity so that parents can 'hear' more clearly and adapt more constructively to the difficult events in their lives. Myers has identified the following characteristics as being important to the success of an interview in terms of maximizing parental wellbeing: the informer should be competent and be aware and comfortable with her own competence and limitations; she should be warm and demonstrate interest in the family and child; she should be patient and accepting of negative responses and be prepared to listen and take into account the parents' point of view; and she should be tolerant of expressions of emotion and also sensitive to feeling states. Myers further stressed that the informer should always be sure to use language that parents can understand and exercise good clinical judgement regarding the amount of information that parents can comprehend, the timing of what is told and the need for further interviews. The ability to be direct and honest when necessary is clearly essential for the occasions when the professional must confront the parents to rectify a misunderstanding.

There are a number of important aspects about the informing interview which warrant discussion. Poor management of the situation has been noted in a number of studies (Pueschel and Murphy, 1976). Privacy is a primary consideration since it allows freedom for the expression of emotions. The literature further advocates that both parents should be present when the diagnosis is first related to the family (Barbor, 1983; Myers, 1983). Indeed, Barbor (1983) has argued that it is difficult for the father to support his wife fully if he gets information secondhand rather than directly from the doctor. Myers (1983) has outlined in some detail what he considers to be good communication skills at the stressful interview and Barbor (1983) has set out a checklist of discussion points — both these articles provide useful guidelines for practice. Lansdown (1980) has also offered advice for professionals.

The importance of good communication between doctors and parents is demonstrated by Johnson, Rudolph and Hartmann (1979), who found that unanswered medical questions were a major source of distress to parents. Further, findings suggest that misunderstanding and disagreement between the professionals and the family may cause seemingly unusual reactions in the patient and family (Mulhern, Crisco and Camitta, 1981).

The Child

Interestingly, a major topic in the early literature was not the reaction of the child to diagnosis but whether the child should be informed of the diagnosis. Two approaches emerged: the protective and the open. This literature is well reviewed by van Dongen-Melman and Sanders-Woudstra (1986), who concluded that a number of carefully controlled studies demonstrated that even young children with cancer are aware of the seriousness of their illness and the threat of death so that an open approach is the most appropriate. Indeed, the literature suggests that children as young as five years may have a good grasp of the meaning of the word 'death'. Lansdown and Benjamin (1985) have argued that if a child appears verbally competent, there is a good chance that even a 4–5-year-old will be able to discuss death in a way that superficial readings of the literature might lead one to imagine unlikely. Lansdown (1985) has cautioned that even some three-year-old children have a greater understanding than anticipated. Koocher (1974) has set out some useful guidelines about how one might talk to children about death. He suggested that for children less than seven years it is most helpful if the explanation is simple and direct, with some reference to personal experience.

Robotham (1983) has argued that, in her own experience, most parents do not wish their child to know the diagnosis and this wish is respected. However, she acknowledged that the amount and accuracy of the information such children acquire through their own means is an unknown quantity. Indeed, Spinetta (1974) has argued that a child as young as six years has a very real awareness of the seriousness of his condition and that reliance upon overt expressions of death anxiety that are easily observed can give a faulty or incomplete picture of the actual anxieties and concerns of the fatally ill child. Swaffield (1985) has suggested that a more open and honest attitude in the care of fatally ill children may be helpful to all concerned since it is apparent that many children know something of their condition without having been told. In an excellent article, Spinetta (1980) described how best to talk to a child about a life-threatening disease while taking into account relevant factors concerning parent and child which may influence this communication.

However, while the literature seems to suggest that the open approach should be employed in every case, both Swaffield (1985) and Spinetta (1978) have emphasized that open communication is not necessarily appropriate in all families in all circumstances. Regarding children's questions, however, as truthful a reply as possible should always be given, indeed, Jolly (1981) has argued that children build up trust with their nurses through good, sensitive communication which is truthful in any information or answers given.

The Needs of the Child during the Illness

The diagnosis of cancer is associated with a life-threatening disease and most children quickly become aware of the seriousness of the disease. This awareness is associated with an increase in anxiety (Spinetta, 1974) and it has been demonstrated that children with cancer experience significantly more anxiety related to the seriousness of their illness than healthy children or children with non-fatal chronic illnesses (Spinetta, Rigler and Karon, 1973). Emotional disturbance has also been found among boys suffering from Duchenne muscular dystrophy (Leibowitz and Dubowitz, 1981); however, Stewart (1984) has argued that much of the emotional strain of having cystic fibrosis may be overcome if the parents have a positive attitude to the child's physical disabilities.

Bluebond-Langer (1978) in her sensitive research demonstrated the different stages of awareness that a child passes through as he gathers a realization of his finite lifespan. She argued that this process was not directly related to the child's age but was rather a function of the child's experience with his disease and its treatment. Thus a four-year-old may have reached the final stage of awareness while an older child still in first remission with limited contact with health professionals and hence less experienced may have passed through the first stages only. Spinetta and Maloney (1975) also found disease experience to be important — they found that children with leukaemia became more anxious with the progression of the disease and with each clinic visit. Further, Lansky and Gendel (1978) observed an extreme separation anxiety with regressive behaviour among children with cancer and, interestingly, the history prior to diagnosis did not suggest such a development.

Medical progress has changed the outlook for many children so that the imminence of death has been replaced by uncertain survival. Indeed, survival is in the context of ever-present doom and the anxiety associated with imminent death is not dispelled (Ably, 1980; Obetz *et al.*, 1980). Robotham (1983) has argued that some of the worst times for child and parent alike are when a relapse occurs; such times frequently reduce both parents and child to the nadir of despair.

The physical discomfort associated with medical treatment to attain remission does not have a place in this chapter, however; suffice it to say that modern treatments are not without side-effects and invariably involve a high degree of acute distress. This literature is well reviewed by van Donger-Melman and Sanders-Woudstra (1986). Another distressing feature of the fatal disease is the necessity of frequent hospitalization as attempts at taming the disease's progress are made. The emotional distress that this causes has been well documented (Bowlby, 1969; Robertson, 1970; Jolly, 1981).

Good nursing care can greatly ameliorate the wellbeing of children during treatment. In particular, Patel (1983) has argued that familiar faces and continuity of care by the same people assist in creating and maintaining an atmosphere of trust. She, like others, has also advocated the use of books and favourite toys as a means of communication. Indeed, much work has been undertaken in this field (Plank, 1971; Petrillo and Sanger, 1972; de Christopher, 1981; Rodin, 1983). Sensitive nursing can also in part compensate for the loss the child suffers in terms of control of daily routine, privacy, relationships with family and friends and control of every aspect of life. In this context, Jolly (1981) has argued that good paediatric nursing involves the care of the child and his whole family. The particular needs of the adolescent with cancer are discussed in Seminars in Oncology Nursing (1986).

The Needs of the Family during the Illness

Impact of diagnosis upon parents has already been discussed. Frequently parents enter a process of anticipatory mourning as they adjust to the potential loss of their child. Interestingly, it seems that the adaptive value of anticipatory mourning is related to time so that there appears to be a minimal time required to complete the process of anticipatory mourning (Townes, Wold and Holmes, 1974). But there also appears to be a maximum time period up to which anticipatory grief has salutary effects so that parents whose child died after a long illness have a poorer adjustment (Rando, 1983).

Inevitably, the life-threatening nature of the disease influences attitudes to parenting. Parents are frequently advised to treat their child normally although it may be argued that such an approach is not possible in the knowledge of a shortened lifespan for their child. Fife (1978), among others, has noted that parents tend to overprotect and indulge their sick child. Health workers clearly have a function in guiding and supporting parents in their difficult role which involves emotional as well as practical burdens.

It is obvious that rearing a child with a life-threatening disease makes extra demands on parenting skills — talking to the child about the disease and its treatment, supporting the child, taking care of the child's physical condition and preparing the child for death as well as for living. Stewart (1984) has outlined the many adjustments which families have to make in order to cope with the demands of the treatment programme, indeed Butler (1984) has noted that the maintenance of normal family life is invariably thwarted by treatment demands and outpatient appointments. .In a questionnaire survey, Turk (1964) found that the demands on parents made them feel that there was less time for themselves and for their own activities. Stewart (1984) concluded that the cost to families was enormous, and since most treatment depends upon the mother, if she has been working she will have to give up work and assume the full-time responsibility for promoting her child's survival. Cooke and Lawton (1984) also found that within families mothers bear the major burden of child care together with home-making, and that families with a chronically sick/ disabled child generally do not receive much support from relatives, friends and neighbours. The contribution of health professionals is therefore of paramount importance although, sadly, the literature indicates that professional support is frequently found wanting (Fillmore, 1981). Perhaps it is this lack of professional support which in part explains the higher incidence of marital disharmony, as parental relationships are tested to the full so that already existing frictions are exposed.

Amelioration of distress requires that parents are provided with practical help, information and emotional support. The giving of emotional support is perhaps the most difficult task for health professionals because childhood should not be associated with ill-health and distress. Robotham (1983) has emphasized how difficult it is to teach parents to take each day as it comes, and in so doing enjoy the time they have with their children. The holistic approach to care is advocated by Thompson (1985) so that parents become equal partners in the child's care and therefore do not feel bereft of a contribution to their child's wellbeing. The concept of family-centred care is fully explained by Jolly (1981) and emphasizes the importance of maintaining and nurturing family life so that sick children may benefit from expert medical and nursing care whilst still enjoying the benefit of the support offered by their families.

The needs of siblings are easily overlooked. Thompson (1985) has argued that families need to be helped to maintain a balance between the needs of the sick child and other family members, and indeed, the needs of siblings must never be underestimated. The main focus of the literature has been on the sick child and the parents to the neglect of other family members. The parents' preoccupation with the fatally ill child invariably means that the other children receive less attention, a point developed by Lindsay and MacCarthy (1974). In a study, Lavigne and Ryan (1979) found that siblings of chronically ill children were more likely to show symptoms of irritability and social withdrawal than their contemporaries with healthy siblings. The most commonly noticed feelings among siblings are those of jealousy and guilt. This is not surprising since siblings will be aware that their parents treat the ill child differently and, in comparison, they are neglected. Spinetta (1981) has suggested that strengthening parents' awareness of the needs of siblings will result in greater support for them.

Relationships between siblings are complex and cannot be stereotyped. However, children within families frequently have special relationships with each other and, as a consequence, often will have a greater rapport with their sick sibling than their parents. Indeed, Cairns *et al.* (1979) found very similar amounts of emotional distress between sick children and their healthy siblings and, interestingly, some siblings showed more signs of distress than the sick child. Thompson (1985) has advocated that wherever possible brothers and sisters should be encouraged to spend time at the hospital so that they gain a realistic view as to what goes on there. She has asserted that with parents' aid, the nursing staff can help educate the siblings about the disease and confront any fantasies they may have. Such an approach exemplifies the meaning of family-centred care.

The Final Illness

The child approaching death poses an immense challenge to health care workers. Jolly (1981) has argued that the main need of the dying child is for the staff to become sensitive to his feelings, to be truthful in any information they give and, most importantly, to have and make time to listen to what the child wants to say. Kubler-Ross (1983) and Bluebond-Langer (1978) both emphasized dying children's need of sharing their knowledge about death and their need for emotional and physical proximity with their parents.

Kohler and Radford (1985) in a small interview study found that most parents were glad to have had their child at home for terminal care — they felt they were carrying out their child's wishes, while also keeping the family together and maintaining more control of the situation. However, misconceptions by parents concerning addiction or overdose meant that some children had suffered pain needlessly because of parental reluctance to increase the daily dose of analgesia. They have advocated close collaboration with the general practitioner in order to avoid these misunderstandings. However, it is worth noting that general practitioners on average see one child with malignant disease every 25 years, so it is unlikely that they will be familiar with current management (Barbor, 1983) and, further, surveys in general practice regarding adults have revealed that social service support is sometimes lacking (Keane, Gould and Millard, 1983) and that night nursing and home help services frequently fail to meet the needs of patients (Woodbine, 1982). Kohler and Radford (1985) also found the meeting of practical needs in terms of equipment delivery left families feeling frustrated and bitter. However, they found that for most parents the main burden of terminal care at home was psychological and they have advocated a comprehensive preparation for bereavement.

Martinson (1983) has argued that the most appropriate way of caring for a dying child is to sustain the family at home where there is comfort and natural care. This reflects current knowledge that most children do not like hospital and find the environment alien and threatening. Martinson has outlined the philosophy behind good terminal care — comfort care which includes effective pain control and other measures to prevent and control physical discomfort. Aspects of good nursing care are discussed by Copperman (1983), who also emphasizes the necessity of good comfort care as well as sensitivity to the child's perspective. The great emotional need for the proximity of family members is clearly more easily met if a child is nursed at home and, further, it promotes a more normal family life, which is important both for the dying child and for his siblings. A moving account by Cotton, Cotton and Goodall (1981) outlines the benefit of a child's terminal care at home to the other children in the family. It is clear that the siblings greatly benefited from their involvement in the preparations for their brother's death.

However, the provision of good nursing support for children who die at home is not always easy (Smith and Francy, 1982). The family needs much support and help, especially when they have to make difficult decisions. A successful Australian scheme which achieves good home support for dying children and their families is described by Bryan (1984). However, Bennett (1984) found that home care for her 16-month-old son was beset with difficulties which included a lack of communication between health care professionals, an uncertainty in the management of pain control and an inexperience in paediatric terminal care. She suggested an improved system of communication between health professionals so that her particular experience could be avoided in the future. The importance of good communication is also emphasized by Renshaw (1979), who has argued that nurses have an important role to play with parents of dying children due to their ability to offer support in the context of nurse–patient–family conversations — she can therefore act as a sounding board, a comforter and a counsellor.

The hospice movement is well established in the United Kingdom. However, Helen House in Oxford was the first hospital to cater for the special needs of children and is the only hospice of its kind in England, which means that for many families there is no real alternative between hospital and home care. The aims of Helen House have been described by Copsey (1981) and Dominica (1982) began its work in November 1982. During the first year it provided care for 52 children with terminal illness, progressive and incurable illness and very severe handicap (Burne, Dominica and Baum, 1984). The care in Helen House is reflective of the work of hospices generally and priority is given to the relief of distress (physical, emotional, social and spiritual). Hunt (1986) has reviewed the work of Helen House. As time has passed, the number of children travelling long distances to stay at Helen House has increased, suggesting that the needs of these families are not being met by more local provisions. It is interesting that only a very small number of children coming to Helen House do so for symptom control and terminal care rather the resolution of care problems for children attending for respite care is a greater focus of staff time. Out of a total of 120 children who have stayed at Helen House since its opening, 46 had died up to February 1986 (eighteen at Helen House, seventeen at home, ten in hospital, one at boarding school). Another important aspect of this hospice's work is the continued support of the bereaved; the staff maintain contact with all the bereaved families as long as they wish it.

The literature emphasizes the vital role the nurse can play in helping and supporting families when they are facing the impending death of a loved one (Atkin, 1981; Jolly, 1981; Robbins, 1983; Lovell, 1984; Ross-Alaolmolki, 1985). Indeed, Ross-Alaolmolki (1985) has argued that the nurse has an important role through facilitating open channels of communication between the child who is dying, the parents and the health care workers. Yet, in a study Hinds (1985) found that families caring for cancer patients at home needed not only greater assistance with the physical care of patients but also greater psychological support, in particular a place or person to whom they could turn to discuss their fears. However, if Fillmore's (1981) account of professional withdrawal is a reality, the needs of parents and families will continue to be unmet at a time of great crisis.

Bereavement

The death of a child is a devastating experience for the family. Binger *et al.* (1969) reported a high incidence (50 per cent) of emotional disturbance in at least one family member after the child's death. Interestingly, Miles (1985) found no significant difference between parents who had lost children through accidental death or chronic disease. Rather, she found that parents who had higher concurrent life stresses and who were of lower socioeconomic status were at greater risk of emotional symptomatology. Although the expression of grief may alter with the lapse of time, its intensity may not diminish as is generally assumed. Studies have shown that families can experience ongoing difficulties in coping with the loss (Rando, 1983). Indeed, some personal accounts make very poignant reading and emphasize just how traumatic the death of a child can be to some families (Davies, 1981; Malcolm, 1985). It is a mistake to believe that parents 'get over' the loss of their child or that other children in the family compensate for the one who has died (Clench, 1983). Clench has suggested that it takes parents several years to cope with the overwhelming sense of sadness at the loss; however, the time needed for this adjustment is variable.

Newton, Bergin and Knowles (1986) interviewed bereaved parents in an attempt to review the quality of the care provided to these families. While this exercise only represents the experience of a very small number of families (twelve), it is worthy of comment because it may reveal a number of weaknesses in the delivery of care. Newton *et al.* have advocated that follow-up interviews should be extended to all families because such an opportunity provides not only a chance for the doctor to participate in the bereavement counselling process, but also a forum where communication that previously has been poor can be improved — explanation can be improved on and misapprehension dispelled. Further, it provides parents with the opportunity to discuss their views and offer personal thanks if they so wish. Kohler and Radford (1985) also identified unmet needs among bereaved parents and stated that a greater commitment was needed to support bereaved families. Two reports have demonstrated how postmortem family support in the context of perinatal and sudden infant death can be effective and reduce morbidity (Forrest, Standish and Baum, 1982; Woodward et al., 1985).

Mina (1985) also found a weakness in the support of bereaved parents. She commented that the nurses provided excellent physical care but only some were able to provide emotional support, and indeed, some nurses hesitated to mention the loss at all. Interestingly, the nurses had also expressed the wish that they could do more to help parents and this perhaps reflected the finding that most of the parents expressed a wish to learn more about the loss and grieving process. A perinatal loss programme was established with success and it was noted that the programme not only helped bereaved parents but also improved staff job satisfaction.

Lack of good support at the time of death of a child is a consistent theme in the literature and emphasizes the need for improved professional education. Liddell (1982) has argued that the training for counselling has not been as beneficial as expected because of its emphasis upon what to say rather than on how to listen. As a consequence, counsellors often fail to hear parents' pleas, which means that parents are not helped in their resolution of confused feelings and are therefore handicapped in the support they are able to give the dying child and other family members. Waters (1982) has similarly argued that while conscientious nursing care is important, it is not always what is done for the family but rather how it is done which counts. Indeed, the quality of communication is considered by Hacking (1981) to be the basis of good care. She has argued cogently that nurses are able to prepare families for the loss of their loved one and to continue to offer support appropriately after the death of a family member. In performance of this role, nurses and other workers need to be mindful of the evidence that families with dying children frequently suffer professional withdrawal (Fillmore, 1981).

There are several organizations which can help parents, for example CRUSE, the Compassionate Friends and the National Association for the Welfare of Children in Hospital. However, none of these groups can take the place of good communication between professionals and parents and it is easy to overlook the continuing needs of families after the death of their child. Collinge and Stewart (1983) have emphasized that many parents may require help and support for many months. Indeed, they have quoted the remarks of a bereaved parent in which she described her profound sense of loneliness and isolation and her increased feelings of emotional pain after the loss of her child. One hospital provides a support booklet for parents in an attempt to help parents come to terms with their loss (Goodall, 1984).

As with literature concerned with the fatally ill child, the needs of the bereaved child have received limited attention. Benians (1984) has argued that only the very young child (under three months of age) whose physical care remains satisfactory will be unaware of the death of a close relative, and subsequently a child's sense of loss will be proportionate to the importance to him of the person who died. This, of course, reflects increasing age and emotional maturity. However, a child's reaction to the death of a sibling not only depends upon developmental stage, but also individual personality, life experiences and the way in which the event is dealt with by parents and others (Westcott, 1982). Young children find it difficult to differentiate between fact and fantasy and frequently feel responsible for the death and it is important that a child is reassured that the death in no way reflected his previous thoughts or actions, even if he does not mention this feeling of guilt. The bereaved child as well as feeling sad may also feel angry that his sibling has deserted him and will no longer play a part in his life. In view of this, children need to be reassured through touch and in words that they will not be left and abandoned. Benians (1984) has advocated that children should be encouraged to share in the family grieving and even allowed to see the dead body. He has argued that seeing and touching the dead body helps children appreciate the reality of what has happened and helps show how harmless the dead body is. Westcott (1982) has further asserted that because few children now have contact with death, owing to improved mortality rates, the death of a pet provides a good opportunity for the rehearsal of suitable reactions and rituals and for a discussion which will allow children to learn of death as a normal part of everyday life. Indeed, Pincus (1974) has long advocated an early discussion and understanding of death in children.

While most children adjust with time to the loss, some develop abnormal grieving which will require expert professional help. However, there is evidence that sibling death during childhood may have a devastating effect upon children (Balk, 1983). Pettle-Michael and Lansdown (1986) found a high percentage of children were exhibiting emotional or behavioural difficulties or both when interviewed 18–30 months after their sibling's death. Interestingly, they did not find an association between parental and sibling adjustment. In contrast to Benians (1984), they did not advocate that the child should see the dead body because in their study seeing the dead body and the sibling dying at home were more frequently experienced by children having pronounced emotional or behavioural difficulties. They found the following experiences helpful to bereaved children: being informed of the likely fatal outcome, participating in the patient's care, having the opportunity to 'say goodbye' near the time of death, attending the funeral or being with the rest of the family on the day of the funeral, being able to have some of the sibling's possessions, and previously experiencing the death of a pet or relative. Balk (1983) interviewed adolescents subsequent to sibling death and found that most teenagers were adjusting satisfactorily although he emphasized that all had endured considerable stress and that the death was likely to have an enduring influence on their lives — a point developed by Wolff (1981). Huxley-Robinson (1985) has argued that the school nurse can aid children in overcoming the effects of bereavement through skilful counselling, although professional help is unfortunately often reserved for those children manifesting unacceptable behaviour. In an ideal world, she has suggested that all children should be prepared for bereavement and sympathetically counselled and supported after the death.

Conclusion

Death in childhood subsequent to a long illness is a relatively rare occurrence and it is not confined to children who have had a malignant disorder. The diagnosis of a fatal condition in a child has a profound effect upon families and requires sensitive and professional management. The literature suggests that, in most cases, children should be informed of their diagnosis and its meaning to them. Good nursing care of fatally ill children requires not only good physical care, but sensitive emotional support of both the ill child and his whole family. The literature has highlighted the emotional needs of siblings as well as parents, not only during the terminal illness but also subsequent to the death of the child.

Helpful Organizations Mentioned in the Chapter

CRUSE — Cruse House, 126 Sheen Road, Richmond, Surrey, TW9 1UR (telephone: 01–940–4818).

Society of Compassionate Friends — c/o Mrs Hadder, 5 Lower Clifton Hill, Bristol 8 (telephone: 0272–292778).

National Association for the Welfare of Children in Hospital (NAWCH) — 7 Exton Street, London, SE1 8VE (telephone: 01–261–1738).

References

Ably, N. (1980) Ending the chemotherapy of acute leukaemia: a period of difficult weaning. In Schulman, J.L., and Kupst, M.J. (eds) *The Child with Cancer*. Charles C. Thomas, Springfield, Illinois.

Atkin, M.E. (1981) Fatal illness: How does the family cope? *Nursing*, 1009–1011.

Balk, D. (1983) Effects of sibling death on teenagers, *Journal of School Health*, **53** (1), 14–18.

Barbor, P. (1983) Emotional aspects of malignant disease in children, *Maternal and Child Health*, **8** (8), 320–327.

Benians, R. (1984) The bereaved child, *Maternal and Child Health*, **9** (1), 4–8.

Bennett, P. (1984) A care team for terminally ill children, *Nursing Times*, March 7, 26–27.

Binger, C.M., Ablin, A.R., Fellerstein, R.C., Kushner, J.H., Zager, S., and Mikkelson, C. (1969) Childhood leukaemia: Emotional impact on patient and family, *New England Journal of Medicine*, **280**, 414–418.

Bluebond-Langer, M. (1978) *The Private Worlds of Dying Children*. Princetown University Press, New Haven.

Bowlby, J. (1969) *Attachment and Loss, I: Attachment*. Penguin, Harmondsworth.

Bryan, N. (1984) Children who die at home, *Nursing Times. Community Outlook*, May 9, 167–169.

Burne, S.R., Dominica, F., and Baum, J.D. (1984) Helen House — a hospice for children: Analysis of the first year, *British Medical Journal*, **289**, 1665–1668.

Burton, L. (ed.) (1974) *The Care of the Child Facing Death*. Routledge & Kegan Paul, London.

Butler, S. (1984) Helping the family to cope, *Nursing Times. Community Outlook*, November 14, 400–401.

Cairns, N.U., Clark, G.M., Smith, S.D., and Lansky, S.B. (1979) Adaptation of siblings to childhood malignancy, *Journal of Paediatrics*, **95**, 484–487.

Clench, P. (1983) Loss of a child, *Nursing*, **2** (20), 590–591.

Collinge, P., and Stewart, E.D. (1983) Dying children and their families. In Robbins, J. (ed.) *Caring for the Dying Patient and the Family*. Lippincott Nursing Series. Harper & Row, London.

Cooke, K., and Lawton, D. (1984) Informal support for the carers of the disabled child, *Child: Care, Health and Development*, **10** (2), 67–69.

Copperman, H. (1983) Dying at Home. Wiley, Chichester.

Copsey, M.K. (1981) Time to care, *Nursing Mirror*, November 25, 38–40.

Cotton, M., Cotton, G., and Goodall, J. (1981) A brother dies at home, *Maternal and Child Health*, **6** (6), 288–292.

Cowie, V. (1983) An inbuilt tragedy, *Nursing Mirror*, February 23, 48–49.

Davies, J. (1981) Why are you crying? *Community Care*, August 6, 12–13.

de Christopher, J. (1981) Children with cancer: their perceptions of the health care experience, *Topics in Clinical Nursing*, **2** (4), 9–19.

Dodge, J.A. (1974) The size and nature of the problem. In Burton, L. (ed.) *Care of the Child Facing Death*. Routledge & Kegan Paul, London.

Dominica, Mother F. (1982) Helen House — a hospice for children, *Maternal and Child Health*, **7** (9), 355–359.

Dubowitz, V. (1978) Muscle disorders in childhood, W.B. Saunders, London.

Fife, B.L. (1978) Reducing parental overprotection of the leukaemic child, *Social Science and Medicine*, **12**, 117–122.

Fillmore, A. (1981) The dying child and professional withdrawal, *Health Visitor*, **54** (8), 328–330.

Forrest, G.C., Standish, E., and Baum, J.D. (1982) Support after perinatal death: a study of support and counselling after bereavement, *British Medical Journal*, **285**, 1475–1479.

Goodall, J. (1984) Notes for parents who have lost a child, *Maternal and Child Health*, **9** (4), 119–122.

Hacking, M. (1981) Dying and bereavement, *Nursing*, 1168–1170.

Hammond, G.D. (1986) The cure of childhood cancers, *Cancer*, **58** (2), 407–413.

Hinds, C. (1985) The needs of families who care for patients with cancer at home: Are we meeting them? *Journal of Advanced Nursing*, **10**, 575–581.

Hunt, A. (1986) Open house, *Nursing Times*, August 27, 53–57.

Huxley-Robinson, M. (1985) Counselling the bereaved child: the role of the school nurse, *Health Visitor*, **58** (9), 253–255.

Johnson, F.L., Rudolph, L.A., and Hartmann, J.R. (1979) Helping the family cope with childhood cancer, *Psychosomatics*, **20**, 241–251.

Jolly, J. (1981) *The Other Side of Paediatrics*. Macmillan, London.

Keane, W.G., Gould, J.H., and Millard, P.H. (1983) Death in practice, *Journal of Royal College of General Practitioners*, **33**, 347–351.

Kohler, J.A., and Radford, M. (1985) Terminal care for children dying of cancer: Quantity and quality of life, *British Medical Journal*, **291**, 115–116.

Koocher, G.P. (1974) Talking with children about death, *American Journal of Orthopsychiatry*, **44** (3), 404–411.

Kubler-Ross, E. (1983) *On Children and Death*. Macmillan, New York.

Lansdown, R. (1980) *More than Sympathy*. Tavistock, London.

Lansdown, R. (1985) Coping with child death: A child's view, *Nursing*, 1264–1266.

Lansdown, R., and Benjamin, G. (1985) The development of the concept of death in children aged 5–9 years, *Child: Care, Health and Development*, **11** (1), 13–20.

Lansky, S.B., and Gendel, M. (1978) Symbiotic repressive behaviour patterns in childhood malignancy, *Clinical Pediatrics*, **17**, 133–138.

Lavigne, J.V., and Ryan, M. (1979) Psychologic adjustment of siblings with chronic illness, *Pediatrics*, **63**, 616–627.

Leibowitz, D., and Dubowitz, V. (1981) Intellect and behaviour in Duchenne muscular dystrophy, *Developmental Medicine and Child Neurology*, **23**, 577–590.

Liddell, G. (1982) Death of a child, *Nursing*, **1** (34), 1496–1497.

Lindsay, M., and MacCarthy, D. (1974) Caring for the brothers and sisters of a dying child. In Burton, L. (ed.) *Care of the Child Facing Death*, Routledge & Kegan Paul, London.

Lovell, B. (1984) A family affair, *Nursing Mirror*, January 11, 19–21.

Malcolm, D. (1985) Letting Alan go, *Nursing Times*, July 17, 30–31.

Martinson, I. (1983) Care of the dying child — 1, *Nursing Times*, March 16, 56–57.

Mearns, M.B. (1985) Cystic fybrosis, *Archives of Disease in Childhood*, **60**, 272–277.

Miles, M.S. (1985) Emotional symptoms and physical health in bereaved parents, *Nursing Research*, **34** (2), 76–81.

Mina, C.F. (1985) A program for helping grieving parents, *Maternal and Child Nursing*, **10** (2), 118–121.

Mulhern, R.K., Crisco, J.J., and Camitta, B.M. (1981) Patterns of communication among pediatric patients with leukemia, parents and physicians: Prognostic disagreements and misunderstandings, *Journal of Pediatrics*, **99**, 480–483.

Myers, B.A. (1983) The informing interview, *American Journal of Disease in Childhood*, **137**, 572–577.

Newton, R.W., Bergin, B., and Knowles, D. (1986) Parents interviewed after their child's death, *Archives of Disease in Childhood*, **61**, 711–715.

Obetz, S.W., Swenson, W.M., McCarthy, C.A., Gilchrist, G.S., and Burgert, E.O. (1980) Children to survive maligant disease: Emotional adaptation of the children and their families. In Schulman, J.L., and Kupst, M.K. (eds) *The Child with Cancer*. Charles C. Thomas, Springfield, Illinois.

OPCS (1982) *Mortality Statistics*. Her Majesty's Stationery Office, London.

Patel, N. (1983) A big challenge from the small, *Nursing Mirror*, Jan. 5, 29–30.

Petrillo, M., and Sanger, S. (1972) *The Emotional Care of the Hospitalised Child*. Lippincott, Philadelphia.

Pettle Michael, S.A., and Lansdown, R.G. (1986) Adjustment to the death of a sibling, *Archives of Disease in Childhood*, **61**, 278–283.

Pincus, L. (1974) *Death and the Family*. Random House, Pantheon Books, New York.

Plank, E. (1971) *Working with Children in Hospital*, 2nd edn. Press of Case-Western Reserve, Cleveland.

Pueschel, S., and Murphy, A. (1976) Assessment of counselling practices at the birth of a child with Down's Syndrome, *American Journal of Mental Deficiency*, **81**, 325–330.

Rando, T.A. (1983) An investigation of grief and adaptation in parents whose children have died from cancer, *Journal of Pediatric Psychology*, **8**, 3–20.

Renshaw, D.C. (1979) The nurse's role with parents of the dying child. *Journal of Nursing Education*, **18** (1), 17–20.

Robbins, J. (ed.) (1983) *Caring for the Dying Patient and the Family*. Lippincott Manual. Harper & Row, London.

Robertson, J. (1970) *Young Children in Hospital*. Tavistock, London.

Robotham, A. (1983) Children with leukemia, *Nursing Times*, February 16,

28–29.

Rodin, J. (1983) *Will This Hurt?* Royal College of Nursing, London.

Ross-Alaolmolki, K. (1985) Supportive care for families of dying children, *Nursing Clinics of North America*, **20** (2), 457–466.

Seminars in Oncology Nursing (1986) *The Adolescent with Cancer*, **2** (2).

Smith, M.L., and Francy, D. (1982) When a child dies at home, *Nursing (American)*, 66–67.

Spinetta, J.J. (1974) The dying child's awareness of death, *Psychological Bulletin*, **81** (4), 456–460.

Spinetta, J.J. (1978) Communication patterns in families dealing with life-threatening illness. In Sahler, O.J.Z. (ed.) *The Child and Death*. C.V. Mosky, St Louis.

Spinetta, J.J. (1980) Disease-related communication: How to tell. In Kellerman, J. (ed.) *Psychological Aspects of Childhood Cancer*. Charles C. Thomas, Springfield, Illinois.

Spinetta, J.J. (1981) The sibling of the child with cancer. In Spinetta, J.J., and Deasy-Spinetta, P. (eds) *Living with Childhood Cancer*. C.V. Masky, St Louis.

Spinetta, J.J., and Maloney, L.J. (1975) Death anxiety in the outpatient leukemic child, *Pediatrics*, **56**, 1034–1037.

Spinetta, J.J., Rigler, D., and Karon, M. (1973) Anxiety in the dying child, *Pediatrics*, **52**, 841–845.

Stewart, A. (1984) Supporting the parents, *Nursing Times*, May 16, 25–26.

Swaffield, L. (1985) Protecting the parents? *Nursing Times*, July 31, 51–52.

Taylor, D.C. (1982) Counselling the parents of handicapped children, *British Medical Journal*, **284**, 1027–1028.

Thompson, J. (1985) Family centred care, *Nursing Mirror*, February 13, 25–28.

Townes, B.D., Wold, D.A., and Holmes, T.H. (1974) Parental adjustment to childhood leukemia, *Journal of Psychosomatic Research*, **18**, 9–14.

Turk, J. (1964) Impact of cystic fybrosis on family functioning, *Pediatrics*, **34**, 66–71.

van Dongen-Melman, J.E.W.M., and Sanders-Woudstra, J.A.R. (1986) Psychosocial aspects of childhood cancer: A review of the literature, *Journal of Child Psychology and Psychiatry*, **27** (2), 145–180.

Waters, M.J. (1982) The needs of the dying patient and family, *Nursing*, 1477–1478.

Westcott, P. (1982) Death, the last taboo, *Mother and Baby*, March, 26–28.

Wolff, S. (1981) *Children Under Stress*, 2nd edn. Penguin, Harmondsworth.

Woodbine, G. (1982) The care of patients dying from cancer, *Journal of Royal College of General Practitioners*, **32**, 685–689.

Woodward, S., Pope, A., Robson, W.J., and Hagan, O. (1985) Bereavement counselling after sudden infant death, *British Medical Journal*, **290**, 363–365.

Part 4   Coping

Nursing Issues and Research in Terminal Care
Edited by J. Wilson-Barnett and J. Raiman
© 1988 John Wiley & Sons Ltd.

CHAPTER 5

Coping with Dying

SALLY SIMS

Chapter Contents

This chapter discusses how individuals respond to the knowledge of
death and outlines ways in which patient and family coping can be
facilitated. Although much has been written on the impact of death
from psychological, philosophical, sociological and religious perspectives, there have been comparatively few empirical studies on how
individuals respond to and cope with the knowledge of death. Possible
directions for future research are therefore outlined at the end of the
chapter.

Introduction

At no time in history has so much attention been paid to death as a
subject for scholarly, literary and clinical study. The large number of
publications on death and dying attest to this (Simpson, 1979). There
are numerous classical works which have been, and remain, influential
in promoting awareness and understanding of death from a number of
different perspectives (for example Freud, 1917; Fiefel, 1959;
Glaser and Strauss, 1965, 1968; Eissler, 1973; Kastenbaum
and Aisenberg, 1972; Schoenberg *et al.*, 1972). Others have provided
insight through extensive clinical experience (for example Quint, 1967;
Kubler Ross, 1970; Weisman, 1972). Although some of these classical
works will be referred to, they are too numerous to review here in
depth. One common theme to emerge from them will be considered

in detail, however: the importance of psychological care for the dying patient and family.

For the purpose of this discussion, responses to dying and descriptions of emotions characterizing the terminal phase of life can be divided according to two alternative hypotheses:

— Responses to dying comprise a predictable, sequential stress response or 'stages of dying'.
— Responses to dying comprise a non-sequential stress response which reflects the individual's usual pattern of responding to stress.

Although little empirical evidence exists to suggest that one hypothesis has greater validity than the other, general opinion favours the latter. Indeed the incidence, severity and relief of psychological distress among the dying has been poorly researched. Comparatively few systematic observations of individuals' responses to dying have been reported in the literature (Hinton, 1963; Lieberman, 1965; Glaser and Strauss, 1965; Kubler Ross, 1970; Wiesman, 1972) and there is a dearth of nursing research related to the psychological care of the terminally ill. Further research on responses to dying, death concerns and coping with dying is needed, including the systematic comparison and cross-validation of direct and indirect measures.

Responding to Dying — Stages of Dying

Kubler Ross (1970) is the most frequently quoted advocate of a predictable staged response to dying. In her book *On Death and Dying* she describes a five-staged response to dying based on observations of more than 200 dying patients who were interviewed (Table 1).

According to Kubler Ross (1970), the patient's initial response to dying is a temporary state of shock. This is gradually replaced by the first distinct stage, denial. In the latest edition of her book, Kubler

Table 1. Stages of dying (Kubler Ross, 1970)

Stage I	Denial
Stage II	Anger
Stage III	Bargaining
Stage IV	Depression
Stage V	Acceptance

Ross (1970) suggests that denial, or at least partial denial, is used by almost all patients, not only pre diagnosis and at the time of diagnosis, but also later from time to time.

There has been much debate about the prevalence and function of the denial of death. It is often assumed, possibly because of an oversimplification of Kubler Ross's (1970) stages, that acceptance of death is desirable and signifies psychological health and that denial does not. Kubler Ross's (1970) earlier work suggested to many that denial and acceptance of death are an 'either/or' reaction; either death is denied or accepted. Weisman (1972) points out that denial and acceptance may exist at the same time, since reason and emotion may conflict. At a conscious level an individual may accept death while at an unconscious level he may deny it. Denial of death is not necessarily negative; it may serve two important functions. Firstly, it may keep the focus away from threatening issues of death and loss and prevent the patient from being overwhelmed (Weisman, 1972) and secondly, it may preserve relationships threatened by the knowledge of terminal illness and prevent social withdrawal from the patient (Beilin, 1981–82). In this way temporary denial can facilitate a more gradual transition to the realization of death. Commonly there is an ambivalent state for which the term 'middle knowledge' has been coined — the individual both recognizes that he is dying and repudiates death (Hackett and Weisman, 1962).

The second response in Kubler Ross's (1970) stages of dying is anger. When denial cannot be maintained any longer Kubler Ross (1970) suggests that it is replaced by feeling of anger, rage, 'why me?'. From the staff and family's point of view this stage may be difficult to cope with, as anger may be projected almost randomly at anyone. Bargaining, the third stage, is relatively brief. The patient believes that he can succeed in entering some sort of agreement which may postpone the inevitable happening. He may offer good behaviour, for example prayer, in return for postponement of death. Once a specific deadline has been reached the patient may, however, begin the process of bargaining over again, asking for more time.

The fourth stage, depression, occurs as a result of anticipated or actual loss, for example loss of role, loss of bodily function, loss of loved ones. According to Kubler Ross (1970), patients should be encouraged to work through their denial, anger and depression and in so doing, reach the final stage of dying, acceptance. Kubler Ross (1970) sees acceptance not as a resigned and hopeless giving up but a state when the patient is neither depressed nor angry about his fate. Towards the end of life Kubler Ross (1970) observed that patients tend to withdraw from all but the most intimate of relationships.

Kubler Ross (1970) completes her description of the stages of dying with the assertion that a little hope runs throughout all of the stages and that patients are aware of the terminal nature of their illness whether or not they have been informed. All patients, according to Kubler Ross, have an opportunity to work through the stages in order to achieve 'a good death' and although some patients reach acceptance without assistance, most need help to do so. She also suggests that family members experience the same stages of adjustment and that if members of a family can share these emotions with each other, they can come to the stage of acceptance together.

A Critique of the Stages of Dying

Kubler Ross's (1970) exposition of the stages of dying has probably been more influential than any other theory in promoting awareness of the psychological needs of the terminally ill; however, her work has received a number of criticisms. Kubler Ross is criticized for being highly subjective; she fails to establish how she identified the stages of dying and appears to have relied on intuition rather than any systematic assessment of responses from the patient (Schulz, 1978). Unless it is possible to identify each of the stages with some degree of certainty, the predictive value of Kubler Ross's (1970) stages of dying is severely impaired. In addition, her theory fails to take into account the significance of age, sex, personality, culture, social background, disease process, environment, previous experience of death and coping ability in the patient's reaction to dying.

Kubler Ross (1970) also fails to present any real evidence to suggest that the same individual actually moves through all stages or that the stages are passed through sequentially (Kastenbaum and Costa, 1977). A small nursing study by Qvarnstrom (1979) casts doubt on the validity of a stage theory of dying. The patients Qvarnstrom (1979) observed did not go through stages but demonstrated an intermingling of responses. In addition to the doubts about the uniformity and progressive nature of Kubler Ross's stages of dying, Carr (1982) points out that it cannot be assumed that an individual needs to negotiate all of the stages in order to cope most effectively with impending death. There is no evidence to suggest that the absence of a specific emotion means that the person has omitted a necessary stage in adjusting to dying or that only acceptance signifies healthy coping.

From a review of a number of studies which have looked at reactions to various stress-producing situations. Falek and Britton (1974) suggest that (1) shock and denial, (2) anger, (3) anxiety and/or guilt and (4) depression are the four responses most commonly observed in individuals under stress. They suggest that these are basic stress reactions or coping responses which are not particular to the trauma but which may be elicited in any situation of severe stress in order to reestablish the steady state.

Indeed, Kubler Ross's (1970) stages of dying are very similar to the phases of mourning put forward by Engel (1962) and Bowlby and Parkes (1979) (Table 2). These similarities do not confirm a stage theory of dying but highlight the normality of disbelief, sadness and anxiety in the face of separation and loss. The same criticisms of Kubler Ross's (1970) stages of dying have been made of the phases of mourning. Worden (1982) does not believe that all individuals pass through all of the phases of mourning or pass through them chronologically. In addition he points out that phases/stages imply that the individuals move passively from one phase/stage to the next. Worden (1982) suggests that the process of accepting the reality of loss and detaching oneself from the lost object (whether it be life or another person) comprises a number of 'tasks' rather than 'stages or phases'.

Table 2. A comparison of the stages of dying and the phases of mourning (after Speck, 1978; by permission of Baillière Tindall Ltd)

Stages of dying Kubler Ross (1970)	Phases of mourning Bowlby and Parkes (1970)	Engels (1962)
Denial	Numbness	Denial
Anger	Anger	
		Developing awareness
Bargaining	Disorganization	
Depression		
Aceptance	Reorganization	Resolution

Tasks imply that individuals can confront what is happening to them and approach the situation actively. Crisis theory has alerted us to the work that individuals have to do in order to master any life crisis (Rapoport, 1970). Poss (1980) suggests that the dying patient's work comprises six problem-solving tasks:

— To become aware of impending death
— To balance hope and fear throughout the crisis
— To make an active decision to reverse physical survival in order to die
— To relinquish responsibility and independence
— To separate the self from former experiences
— To prepare the soul for death

According to Poss (1980), accepting one's dying does not necessarily require work on all six tasks and while engaged in these tasks the patient experiences many emotions. Poss identified the six tasks from the literature on crisis theory and from her own observations. Further empirical research is needed to compare the terminal crisis with other life crises such as the crisis of middle adulthood (Erikson, 1950) and to validate Poss's theory of the 'tasks of dying'.

Responding to Dying — an Individualized Stress Response

Although it would be helpful to be able to predict with accuracy the way in which an individual will respond to the process of dying, it is important not to lose sight of the individual in anticipating responses to dying. Carr (1982) points out that individuals have their own particular views of themselves, their families, their future and death. In addition there are a number of variables which may significantly influence how an individual responds to the knowledge of death. These variables include age, personality, disease process, culture, sex, simultaneously occurring stress situations, past experience with death and coping ability. Many discussions about dying focus on the death-denying attitude of western society. The influence of societal attitudes on responses to dying is also important. Two other important factors which may influence responses to dying are awareness of death and pattern of dying; these warrant further discussion here.

Awareness of Dying

In their classic sociological study of interactions with terminally ill patients, Glaser and Strauss (1965) identified four different levels of death awareness or 'awareness contexts'. These refer to the differing levels of awareness about the patient's impending death which may exist between the patient and other individuals.

— Closed awareness
The patient doesn't recognize his own death although everyone else does.
— Suspected awareness
The patient suspects what others know and attempts to confirm or invalidate his suspicions.
— Mutual pretence awareness
Everyone including the patient is aware that the patient is dying but pretends to the other that he doesn't know.
— Open awareness
Everyone including the patient is aware that the patient is dying and acts on this knowledge openly.

The patient's responses to his own death will be influenced by how much he knows and with what certainty. In the same way, others will guide their actions and responses towards the patient depending upon the level of awareness which exists.

Pattern of Dying

Based on intensive fieldwork in hospitals, Glaser and Strauss (1968) have identified a number of different patterns of dying or 'dying trajectories' which also influence the way in which individuals respond to dying. Deaths may be quick or slow and can be further divided into deaths which are expected or unexpected, where the time of death is certain or uncertain. The quick, unexpected death has surprise as its main feature and the patient may have little opportunity to respond. Where death is expected but the time of death is uncertain, greater anxiety may be aroused than if the approximate time of death is certain. Garfield (1978) suggests that the time of most acute anxiety for the dying patient is in the initial acute phase of dying when the patient is aware of death but uncertain of events, whereas as the individual approaches death anxiety diminishes. No evidence is given in support of this claim, however, and further research is needed to explore the ways in which these different variables influence responses to dying.

Evidence suggests that responses to stressful life events, including death, have a number of common characteristics (Falek and Britton, 1974). Provided reactions such as shock, denial, anger, depression, etc., are not equated with 'ideal', 'necessary' or 'inevitable', an awareness of these emotional responses can help health professionals to provide the types of help and support which may be beneficial. The influence of a number of different variables and the patient's unique personality mean, however, that the individual nature of a patient's response to dying should not be overlooked.

Coping with Dying

Although much has still to be learnt about death concerns and responses to dying, research supports the notion that dying evokes significant emotional distress. When an event is perceived as threatening or stressful, individuals respond with one or more coping strategies in an attempt to reestablish the steady state. Coping is a problem-solving process which if effective brings relief, reward, quiescence and equilibrium and if ineffective results in varying degrees of turmoil, anguish, frustration, despair and suffering (Weisman, 1979a). A distinction can be made between coping style, a relatively enduring aspect of personality, and coping strategies, which are techniques for dealing with threatening events (Lipowski, 1970). Coping strategies may be adaptive or maladaptive and consist of a number of active measures to overcome, and passive aversive measures to avoid or minimize, a recognized problem (Lipowski, 1970). Some common coping strategies which may be used by the patient who is facing life-threatening illness or death include (Weisman, 1979a):

— Seeking more information
— Turning to others for support, sharing concerns and talking with others
— Trying to forget, putting it out of mind, denying
— Distracting by concentrating on other things
— Confronting by taking firm action
— Submitting to the inevitable
— Finding meaning and making the most of life
— Tension-reducing strategies such as drink or drugs
— Blaming oneself

Based on research findings and analyses of patients with cancer, Weisman (1979b) suggests that it is possible to differentiate between patients who are most and least vulnerable in highly stressful situations, including the possibility of death in the near future. Patients who cope most effectively and show the least vulnerability employ active problem-solving strategies. They confront their problems and make their own decisions about coping but seek help and information when needed. Effective copers are more willing to discuss their fears and anxieties and to cooperate with health carers. Their overall attitude is more likely to be optimistic whereas patients who employ passive defending coping techniques show greater vulnerability. These patients typically withdraw and suppress their feelings and anxieties rather than choosing to discuss them. They are inclined to be more compliant by nature, seeking little help or information about their illness, tending to be inflexible in behaviour and pessimistic in outlook. Stedeford (1981) found that couples most at risk of making a poor adjustment in the face of death are the under 40s, especially those with children or parents who need them. Marital problems, isolation or estrangement from the extended family, poor communication and underlying personality disorders were also found to increase a couple's difficulties.

The Importance of Effective Coping

Effective coping and the alleviation of emotional distress enhance quality of remaining life and may divert a crisis reaction. If the patient is not able to mobilize his own internal and external resources successfully and fails to receive adequate support, tension may amount to breaking point causing major disorganization of the individual (Caplan, 1964). Appropriate intervention at the correct time may enable an individual to emerge stronger from the situation. Successful coping with the knowledge of death may therefore result in psychological and personal growth (Lipowski, 1970; Ainsworth-Smith and Speck, 1982) and may even prolong life (Weisman, 1974). Carr (1982) points out that there is increasing evidence to indicate that how an individual reacts to and copes with dying influences the timing of death. Shorter survival time is believed to occur in patients who typically show greater dependence, who deny the severity of their condition and who do not have access to, or do not utilize, supportive social relationships. Although most attention has been focused on the patient's reactions to dying and coping ability, family reactions and coping are equally important. Family members who are themselves coping well may be able to mediate the patient's stress. In addition, the way in which the family copes with the circumstances surrounding death is closely linked to the impact of bereavement on the survivors (Cameron and Parkes, 1983).

Facilitating Coping

Facilitating effective coping for the dying patient and family is therefore important and it is pertinent to consider who should receive psychological assistance. There is a tendency to wait and see who develops serious emotional difficulties and then make a referral to a psychologist, social worker or other member of the health care team. While the practical aspects of care may be planned, psychological aspects of care are less likely to be planned and carried out on the basis of accountable decision-making (Knight and Field, 1981). It is important that patients who are at risk of developing problems are recognized in advance and offered support and assistance before emotional distress becomes severe. In order to do this it is necessary to assess each patient and family individually. Assessment factors to consider include:

— What are the sources of perceived stress/distress?
— How are the patient and family responding to the stresses and how effectively are they coping?
— Are the responses/behaviours a cause for concern?
— What past experiences have the patient and family had in dealing with stress and how did they cope?
— How do age, personality, cultural background and religion influence coping ability?
— What additional resources are available?

Carr (1982) suggests that sources of distress for the dying patient and family are numerous, including:

— Awareness of impending death/bereavement, anticipation of loss
— Frustration and helplessness
— Uncertainty about the future/death fears
— Changes in role and changes in ability
— Physical symptoms/personal suffering

Reactions to dying and coping are not only influenced by psychological but also by physiological and social factors. It is therefore important to assess the patient and family's total needs, since unmet needs such as pain, comfort or privacy will adversely affect coping ability. An individual's normal response to stressful events should also be taken into consideration. Hinton's (1975) research on the influence of personality on reactions to having terminal cancer suggests that the manner in which an individual reacts to dying reflects their previous pattern of handling life's demands. Lipowski (1970) has identified a number of factors which influence a person's ability and mode of coping with ill-health (see Table 3). Although empirical evidence is lacking, these factors may influence how an individual copes with life-threatening illness and approaching death.

Table 3. Determinants of coping with physical illness (Lipowski, 1970)

Intrapersonal factors	Disease related	Environmental
Age	Type, location	Social
Personality	Rate of onset and progression	
Intelligence		
Specific skills	Functional improvement	Spatial
Values/beliefs	Potential reversibility*	
Emotional state		
Cognitive capacity		
Timing of illness in lifecycle		

* The less the degree of reversibility, the more coping resources are challenged.

Current understanding of common responses to threatening events and factors which influence a person's ability to cope with them point to the type of nursing interventions which may be beneficial. Based on Taylor's (1983) theory of cognitive adaption to threatening events, a number of interventions will be outlined. Taylor (1983) suggests that the adjustment process in individuals facing threatening events such as death centres on three processes: (1) the search for meaning (why it has happened and the implications), (2) an attempt to regain mastery, and (3) an effort to enhance one's self-esteem. By influencing one or more of these processes, the following interventions may facilitate coping and cognitive adaption:

Interventions	*Elements of cognitive adaption* (Taylor, 1983)
Effective communication	Search for meaning
Participation in care	Regain mastery
Group support	Enhance self-esteem
Stress reduction techniques	

Effective Communication

Effective communication is the foundation of all therapeutic relationships and counselling techniques aimed at helping patients and their families find meaning with the experience of dying. Concerned support and a caring relationship characterized by trust, empathy and respect are essential in order to provide a safe environment in which individuals facing death can disclose their fears and work through their feelings. Kubler Ross (1970) describes the eagerness of her dying patients to talk about their impending death and the relief experienced when they were allowed to unburden themselves, and Weisman (1974) has shown that patients who can talk about their feelings are less vulnerable in stressful situations. Helping patients to share their feelings may therefore be therapeutic. Studies show, however, that dying patients' commmunication needs often go unheeded (Drummond-Mills, 1983; Quint, 1965; Webster, 1981). There are at least three reasons for this. Health carers may fear a permanent negative reaction from the patient on disclosing the terminal nature of the illness (Glaser and Strauss, 1965) and may feel ill-equipped to communicate effectively with the patient or know how best to help him cope with his emotions (Buckman, 1984).

The communication needs of dying patients and their families are both verbal and non-verbal and range from social interaction on the one hand to information about diagnosis and prognosis and discussion about feelings on the other. Hinton's (1963) research has also shown that many patients facing death show increased religiosity; the patient's communication needs may therefore include discussions about spirituality. Some patients prefer not to know or comprehend all the pertinent facts. Individual preferences for the amount of information disclosed should therefore be respected. For the most part, however, information-giving increases knowledge and understanding and promotes a sense of control, with a resultant decrease in anxiety. Certainly patients who are used to coping by seeking more information about a stressful situation may suffer anguish from lack of information. Poor communication may result in significant distress for the dying patient and family (Stedeford, 1981) whereas good communication can facilitate the expression of thoughts and feelings in such a way as to clarify the situation and assist the individual to make appropriate decisions from the choices available. Although the importance of skilled communication in terminal care is now well recognized, further research is needed to determine the types of communication skills training which are most successful in assisting health professionals to meet the communication needs of dying patients and their families, and the types of psychological support patients and their families find most beneficial. Fielding and Llewelyn (1987) point out that there is considerable need for the development of theory to underlie communication skills training and methods to evaluate its effectiveness.

Participation in Care

When an individual perceives his ability to cope as being greater than the threat which confronts him, there is a sense of personal control and mastery. This is rewarding and associated with positive emotion. Perceived lack of control, on the other hand, leads to negative emotion and is associated with loss of self-esteem. The patient who is dying may already experience a lowered self-esteem due to altered body image and feelings of worthlessness. Persistent lack of control where the individual perceives that he is unable to influence demands or outcomes leads to feelings of depression and helplessness (Seligman, 1975). All too often when someone is dying well-meaning individuals move in and take control. It is important that health carers involve the patient and family and that the patient is encouraged to participate in decision-making, as this can facilitate feelings of control. Not everyone will wish to be involved in the care-giving process, but research indicates that in the hospital setting patient and family participation is minimal even by those who would appreciate it and find it beneficial (Brooking, 1982).

Participation in care and self-reliance can enhance feelings of control. It is essential, however, that patient and family receive adequate information and instruction so that they feel confident in this role. Grobe, Ilstrup and Ahrmann's (1981) study of the skills needed by family members to maintain the care of an advanced cancer patient at home indicates that carers do not always receive the information they require. They found that over two-thirds of the respondents reported the need for more information concerning at least one of the following — ambulation, bowel management, comfort skills, diet, pain management, wound and skin care. Patients may suffer additional anxiety if they are concerned about how their relatives are coping. Dubrey and Terrill (1975) found that the majority of dying patients in their study were concerned about their relatives' ability to cope. Further studies are needed to determine which factors influence the participation of terminally ill patients and their families in the care-giving process and to decide on the information required.

Group Support

A number of authors have described the benefits of support groups for patients who are terminally ill and their families (Yalom and Greaves, 1977; Spiegel and Yalom, 1978; Kopel and Mōck, 1978; Spiegel, Bloom and Yalom, 1981). Spiegel and Yalom (1978) suggest that there are a number of beneficial features of group support which are not available from individual therapy, including:

— Universality, the sense that group members are all in the same position
— Altruism, the experience which emerges through helping others
— Instillation of hope; group members can see others who have had similar problems and have coped
— Group cohesiveness, which can offset some of the isolation patients experience.

Spiegel, Bloom and Yalom (1981) disconfirm the view that patients will be demoralized by associating with patients in the same situation. Their evaluation of weekly supportive group meetings for women with metastatic cancer suggests that supportive group intervention can help to develop a sense of mastery. Evidence from American nurses who have run support groups for cancer patients and their families also suggests that this kind of intervention may be beneficial (Miller and Nygren, 1978; Fredette and Beattie, 1986).

Stress Reduction Techniques

A number of techniques exist which enable voluntary control to be exerted over the body's response to stressful events. These include transcendental meditation, relaxation, yoga, guided imagery and biofeedback. The source of stress is not eliminated but the stress response is reduced to a more tolerable level and a sense of mastery may be facilitated (see Chapter 8 — Complementary Therapies as Nursing Interventions).

Directions for Future Research

Individual responses to dying are complex and an eclectic approach to future research is needed if this complexity is to be captured. Although much has been written on death and dying, there are still gaps in our knowledge of the psychological impact of dying. Concomitantly there are gaps in our knowledge concerning the type and range of interventions the dying patient and his family may find most helpful. Further research is needed in both areas by psychological, medical and nursing staff. Directions for future nursing research include studies:

— To compare responses to dying with responses to other life crises
— To establish criteria against which patients and families most at risk of psychological distress can be assessed
— To determine the problems dying patients and their families find most difficult to cope with
— To determine which factors influence patient and family coping with dying, in both hospital and community settings
— To determine the relationship between family coping and patient coping
— To evaluate the effect of specific nursing interventions such as counselling and relaxation training on perceived coping.

References

Ainsworth-Smith, I., and Speck, P. (1982) *Letting Go — Caring for the Dying and Bereaved*, Chapter 1. SPCK.

Beilin, R. (1981–82) Social functions of denial of death, *Omega*, **12** (1), 25–35.

Bowlby, J., and Parkes, C.M. (1970) Separation and loss. In Anthony, E., and Koupernik, C. (eds) *The Child in His Family*, Vol. 1, *International Yearbook of Child Psychiatry and Allied Professions*. Wiley, New York.

Brooking, J. (1982) *Patient and Family Participation in Nursing: A Survey of Opinions, Current Practice among Patients, Relatives and Nurses*, Proceedings of the RCN Research Paper XIII Annual Conference, UK Royal College of Nursing.

Buckman, R. (1984) Breaking bad news: Why is it still so difficult? *British Medical Journal*, **288**, (6430), 1597–1599.

Cameron, J., and Parkes, C.M. (1983) Terminal care: Evaluation of effects on surviving family of care before and after bereavement, *Postgraduate Medical Journal*, **59**, 73–78.

Caplan, G. (1964) *Principles of Preventative Psychiatry*. Tavistock, London.

Carr, A.T. (1982) In Hall, J. (ed.) *Psychology for Health Professionals*, Chapter 17. Macmillan, London.

Drummond-Mills, W. (1983) Problems related to the nursing management of the dying patient. MSc Thesis, University of Glasgow.

Dubrey, R., and Terrill, L. (1975) The loneliness of the dying patient: An exploratory study, *Omega*, **6** (4), 357–371.

Eissler, K. (1973) *The Psychiatrist and the Dying patient*. International University Press, New York.

Engel, G. (1962) *Psychological Development in Health and Disease*. W.B. Saunders, Philadelphia.

Erikson, E. (1950) *Childhood and Society*. W.W. Norton, New York. Revised edition Penguin Books, Harmondsworth, 1965.

Falek, A., and Britton, S. (1974) Phases in coping: The hypothesis and its implications, *Social Biology*, **21** (1), 1–7.

Fiefel, H. (1959) *The Meaning of Death*. McGraw-Hill, New York.

Fielding, R.G., and Llewelyn, S.P. (1987) Communication training in nursing may damage your health and enthusiasm. Some warnings, *Journal of Advanced Nursing*, **12** (3), 281–290.

Fredette, S., and Beattie, H. (1986) Living with cancer: A patient education programme, *Cancer Nursing*, **9** (6), 308–315.

Freud, S. (1917) *Mourning and Melancholia*, Standard edition, Vol. XIV. Hogarth Press, London, 1957.

Garfield, C. (1978) *Psychosocial Care of the Dying Patient*. McGraw-Hill, New York.

Glaser, B., and Strauss, A. (1965) *Awareness of Dying*. Aldine, Chicago.

Glaser, B., and Strauss, A. (1968) *Time for Dying*. Aldine, Chicago.

Grobe, M., Ilstrup, D., and Ahrmann, D. (1981) Skills needed by family members to maintain the care of an advanced cancer patient, *Cancer Nursing*, October, 371–375.

Hackett, T., and Weisman, A. (1962) In Fitzpatrick, R., Hinton, J., Newman, S., Scambler, G., and Thompson, J. (1984) *The Experience of Illness*, Chapter 11. Tavistock, London.

Hinton, J. (1963) The physical and mental distress of the dying, *Quarterly Journal of Medicine*, **XXXII** (125), 1–21.

Hinton, J. (1975) The influence of previous personality on reactions to having terminal cancer, *Omega*, **6** (2), 95–111.

Kastenbaum, R., and Aisenberg, R. (1974) *The Psychology of Death*. Springer, New York.

Kastenbaum, R., and Costa, P. (1977) Psychological perspectives on death, *Ann. Rev. Psychology*, **28**, 225–249.

Knight, M., and Field, D. (1981) A silent conspiracy. Coping with dying cancer patients on an acute surgical ward, *Journal of Advanced Nursing*, **6**, 221–229.

Kopel, K., and Mōck, L. (1978) The use of group sessions for the emotional support of families of terminal patients, *Death Education*, **1**, 409–422.

Kubler Ross, E. (1970) *On Death and Dying*. Tavistock, London.

Lieberman, M. (1965) Psychological correlates of impending death: Some preliminary observations, *Journal of Gerontology*, **20**, 181–190.

Lipowski, Z.J. (1970) Physical illness, the individual and the coping process, *Psychiatry in Medicine*, **1** (3), 91–102.

Miller, S., and Nygren, M. (1978) Preparing the family to care for the cancer patient at home: A home care course, *Cancer Nursing*, Feb., 49–52.

Poss, S. (1980) How the terminal patient accepts dying, *Patient Counselling and Health Education*, **2** (2), 72–77.

Quint, J.C. (1965) Institutionalised practices of information control, *Psychiatry*, **28** (2), 119–132.

Quint, J. (1967) *The Nurse and the Dying Patient*. Macmillan, New York.

Qvarnstrom, U. (1979) Patients' reactions to impending death, *International Nursing Review*, **26** (4), 117–119.

Rapoport, L. (1970) Cited in Poss, S. (1980) How the terminal patient accepts dying, *Patient Counselling and Health Education*, **2** (2), 72–77.

Schoenberg, B., Carr, A., Peretz, D., and Kutscher, A. (1972) *Psychological Aspects of Terminal Care*. Columbia University Press.

Schulz, R. (1978) *The Psychology of Death, Dying and Bereavement*. Addison Wesley, New York.

Seligman, M. (1975) *Helplessness: On Depression Development and Death*. Freeman, San Francisco.

Simpson, M. (1979) *Dying, Death and Grief. A Critically Annotated Bibliography and Source Book of Thanatology and Terminal Care*. Plenum, New York.

Speck, P. (1978) *Loss and Grief in Medicine*. Baillière Tindall, London.

Spiegel, D., and Yalom, I. (1978) A support group for dying patients. *International Journal of Group Psychotherapy*, **28**, 233–245.

Spiegel, D., Bloom, J., and Yalom, I. (1981) Group support for patients with metastatic cancer, *Arch. Gen. Psychiatry*, **38**, 527–533.

Stedeford, A. (1981) Couples facing death. I Psychosocial aspects, *British Medical Journal*, October 17, 1033–1036.

Taylor, S. (1983) Adjustment to threatening events. A theory of cognitive adaptation, *American Psychologist*, Nov., 1161–1173.

Toynbee, A., *et al.* (1968) *Man's Concern with Death*. Hodder & Stoughton, London.

Webster, M. (1981) Communicating with dying patients, *Nursing Times*, **77** (22), 999–1002.

Webster, M. (1986) Care of the dying — easing emotional distress, *Nursing Times*, **82** (44), 43–44.

Weisman, A. (1972) *On Dying and Denying. A Psychiatric Study of Terminality*. Behavioural Publications, New York.

Weisman, A.D. (1974) In Weisman, A.D. (1979) A model for psychosocial phasing in cancer, *General Hospital Psychiatry*, 187–195.

Weisman, A. (1979a) *Coping with Cancer*. McGraw Hill, New York.

Weisman, A. (1979b) A model for psychosocial phasing in cancer, *General Hospital Psychiatry*, 187–195.

Worden, J.W. (1982) *Grief Counselling and Grief Therapy*. Tavistock, New York.

Yalom, I., and Greaves, C. (1977) Group therapy with the terminally ill, *American Journal of Psychiatry*, **134** (4), 396–400.

Nursing Issues and Research in Terminal Care
Edited by J. Wilson-Barnett and J. Raiman
© 1988 John Wiley & Sons Ltd.

CHAPTER 6

Coping with Distressing Symptoms

MARY THOMAS

Introduction

One of the fundamental features of good terminal care is the provision of a 'quality of life'. This has been described as an abstract and complex term derived from the individual's response to physical, mental and social factors (Holmes and Dickerson, 1987). The concept includes a wide variety of characteristics whose inclusion in the planning of care contributes to an holistic approach — which is much written of in terminal care — the 'hospice philosophy' (Manning, 1984; Corr and Corr, 1983).

The challenge of this chapter, reviewing the nursing implications of physically distressing symptoms other than pain, relates to the very nature of nursing itself. Literature relates to the medical model or provides a description of a process of care — however, the question arises should we view clinical phenomena from a different perspective (Carrieri and Lindsey, 1986)?

The value of such a 'conceptual approach' is that it may allow us to assess, plan and evaluate care across disease processes. Within terminal care this is beginning, as practices related to the management of the patient with advanced cancer become generalized to other diseases. Terminal care provides an exciting opportunity for concepts encompassing malignant and non-malignant disease to be developed. Once agreed, these concepts could provide a focus for communication of ideas and research. It may well be that for reasons stated later the hospice movement could act as such a focus.

Other support for this 'conceptual approach' evolves from a study of self-reported distressing symptoms in patients with both malignant and non-malignant disease, in general wards, where links were identified between symptoms (Hockley, 1983). A symptom distress scale was designed to quantify as well as give a value to the quality of distress experienced by the individual patient with cancer (McKorkle and Young, 1978). It is of interest that in a recent study (Holmes and Dickerson, 1987) some symptoms were not 'readily apparent', and thus the nurse or close family may not be aware of the problem, supporting the value of using the above scale or 'quality of life' self-assessment. Hockley's (1983) study identified sixteen major distressing symptoms (see Figure 1).

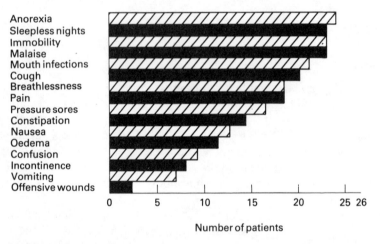

Figure 1. Summary of symptoms reported by patient to researcher. Reproduced from Hockley (1983) by permission of Miss J. Hockley

The following were suggested as areas of teaching needs for families managing patients with advanced disease (Grobe, Ilstrup and Ahman, 1981):

1. Ambulation
2. Bowel management
3. Comfort
4. Diet
5. Pain
6. Wound and skin care

Relief of physical discomfort and relief of physiological responses are seen as a priority by nursing staff (White, 1972). It is interesting that intervention, however, is not always a physical one as other strategies are involved (White, 1972; Sims, 1986; Kershaw and Salvage, 1986).

Roy's stress adaptation model gives a theoretical framework within which to view nursing practice in terminal care (Kershaw and Salvage, 1986). Her philosophy encompasses an holistic approach — 'human beings are biopsychosocial individuals responding to influencing factors from a constantly changing environment using both innate and acquired mechanisms' (Riehl and Roy, 1980). The goal of the nurse is to help people adjust to their position on a health illness continuum and this chapter uses Roy's framework while reviewing the data.

Maybe the apparent dearth of material that has emanated from the hospice movement related to nursing management is linked to its philosophy. Does the scientific method embrace the 'individual approach', fragmentation *versus* allopathy?

If modern terminal care is compared with the development of oncology nursing research then it may suggest areas for future review. It is a priority that designs are sensitive to the rights of the dying patient and his family and, as Petrosino has suggested, 'be viewed very positively by both parties'. Below is a list of physical symptoms organized into a series of concepts which can form the basis for investigation.

Selected examples of these will be reviewed here.

1. Cachexia
2. Anorexia
3. Oedema
4. Pain
5. Impaired sleep
6. Impaired elimination
7. Fatigue
8. Dyspnoea
9. Impaired wound healing

Anorexia

Loss of appetite, or loss of the physiological desire to eat even where there is a clear need for nourishment, is identified by terminally ill patients as the most distressing symptom (Hockley, 1983). Sixty-eight per cent of the patients referred to Strathcarron Hospice were identified as having this problem. Twycross notes that the term anorexia is commonly misused to cover inadequate food intake (Twycross and Lack, 1986, Ch.3), which he discusses as oligophagia. This concept can be studied across disease processes, e.g. in advanced renal disease associated with uraemia, food aversions; in cardiac disease where anorexia is the effect of oedema around the gastrointestinal organs; in advanced cancer where it may be related to abnormalities in taste change, abnormality in glucose metabolism, imbalance of certain amino acids, delayed digestion or mechanical effects — 'squashed stomach syndrome'. It is significant that psychological stress and emotional state will also have a marked impact on dietary intake (Holland, Rowland and Plumb, 1977).

Anorexia in the Terminally Ill

Influencing Factors

    Presence of pain
    Fatigue
    Nausea and vomiting
    Altered taste
        Recent treatment to gastrointestinal system, e.g. surgery, radio-
        therapy
    Mouth problems
    Electrolyte imbalance, water balance

Regulator Mechanisms

Food accumulation in the stomach will inhibit appetite stimulation (Holland, Rowland and Plumb, 1977), while elevated lactic acid levels associated with some tumours will do the same (Schnipper, 1985).

Cognator Factors

Anxiety and depression may significantly affect eating, with stress causing the release of catecholamines.

Behaviour Modes

Pleasure associated with eating is obviously a major goal and it is important to look at individuals' attitude to food — to relieve them from too much pressure from their families to eat. Also the family themselves may need to be 'relieved of their guilt' if they feel they are failing. It is important to respond to individual need but also remain consistent. Mills reports in her observational study that a special dietary item received great attention; however, when the regular meal arrived the patient received little help to eat it (Mills, 1983).

Nursing Intervention

This will include assessment, explanation and teaching. Small meals, provided more frequently and including special preferences, are needed. Food should be provided when requested and presented attractively on small plates. Eating is a social activity, and it is important to be comfortable, pain-free, have a fresh mouth and be provided with all the physical aids that will enhance your feeling of independence. Time is essential. Schnipper describes anorexia as whimsical, i.e. what may work once may not be successful when tried a second time. In conjunction with the management of taste changes and dealing with mouth problems, it is important to remember that the therapeutic use of oral steroids will enhance appetite. The questions must be — what are 'realistic goals' and how can we help our patients and their families to achieve them?

Mouth Problems

There is a large challenge in maintaining good oral hygiene in those who are too ill, depressed or drugged to do it for themselves. Mouths are needed to eat, communicate verbally, and express emotion. Anything therefore interfering with the mouth's normal healthy function is at the least embarrassing, and at worst so painful that eating/drinking/swallowing and talking become difficult or impossible. The main problems to be considered are 'dirty' mouth, pain and dryness. Most patients suffering from a prolonged debilitating illness are subject to any, or all of these. The all too familiar picture of a frail, dependent, apathetic patient, with dry mouth, coated tongue and cracked lips, is well known to us all. His self-image is virtually at its lowest. He is beyond caring that his mouth is in such a condition and resents attempts to improve matters. The motivation to clean his teeth or hydrate himself is gone, as well, perhaps, as the physical ability to do so. It may all seem trivial when measured against a major disease process, but in many instances it appears from the patient's point of view to be the pinnacle of his distress. For example, even kissing may be a

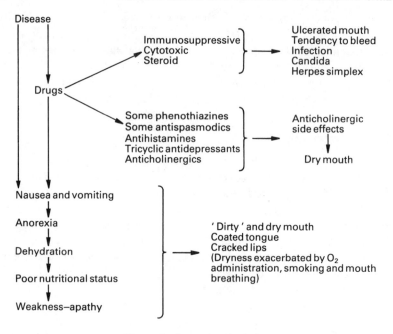

Figure 2. Sore mouth cycle

problem because of the pain of an ulcerated mouth or the shame of halitosis. These factors are interrelated in Figure 2.

Cleaning — why?

Lack of the usual movements of the mouth in chewing and swallowing leads to the formation of plaque as the resulting accumulation of food debris is unable to be cleared without satisfactory salivation. This creates inflammation and irritation of the oral mucosa. A coated tongue is the end result of old epithelial cells, dried mucus and saliva.

With what? (see Table 1)

Glycerine of thymol tastes good but does little other than refresh the mouth. Hydrogen peroxide made into a solution with warm water or normal saline detaches dead tissue and bacteria but does not penetrate a coated tongue. Sodium bicarbonate is cheap and effective. It neutralizes bacterial activity by producing a base alkali, but again is ineffective as regards a furred tongue. Corsodyl is a chlorhexidine preparation with antifungal and antibacterial properties. It inhibits

Table 1. Different cleaning procedures for those with painful or dry mouths

Pain	Dryness
Cause	
Ulcerations and/or infection	Very difficult to treat, likely to be needed 1–2 hourly
Remedy	*Suggestions*
Bland diet — avoid hot, acidic and spicy foods (Daeffler and Daeffler, 1986)	Frequent, careful, oral cleaning (stimulates saliva flow)
Orabase applied topically	Hydrate
Benadryl elixir (Bersani and Carl, 1983)	Small quantities often of 'wet food'
Xylocaine viscous mouthwashes prior to meals (Lane and Forgay, 1981)	Artificial saliva (can be delivered in pray form — Glandosane)
Benzocaine lozenges	
Corsodyl mouthwash	
Betadine mouthwash	Ice-cold drinks at hand
Nystatin solution	Ice cubes, fizzy drinks and chunks
Ketonidazole tablets	of fruit
Natural yoghurt	Vaseline to lips or KY jelly
Idosydidine	Antiherpetic agents for topical
Zovrax ointment	application in herpes simplex

plaque formation, is well tolerated and effective. To merely keep the mouth moist and clean and intact, normal saline or saline/water mouthwashes are useful (Hallett, 1984).

How?

It is preferable to provide a basic mouthwash once dentures have been removed and cleaned and/or teeth brushed, if possible using a small-headed, soft-bristled tooth brush (Bersani and Carl, 1983). Toothpaste such as Sensodyne could be used for sensitive gums. If a toothbrush is not possible, foam sticks, moist swabs on a finger, or gentle irrigation with a Higginson's syringe (so long as the swallowing reflex is intact) could be used (Hallett, 1984).

Taste change — 'the blind mouth'

If taste is not normal this will reduce the desire to eat. This has been demonstrated in cancer patients (de Wyss and Walteresk, 1975). What then is the impact of a 'blind mouth' on the terminally ill?

Studies relating to cancer patients show there is no link with a particular type of neoplasm (de Wyss and Walters, 1975). However, the more advanced the disease, the more apparent the taste change (de Wyss and Walters, 1975). (See Table 2.)

The normal desire to eat is achieved by having a functioning sense of taste and smell and it is suggested that 25–50 per cent of this may be affected (Twycross and Lack, 1986, p. 59).

Attacking oral hygiene problems is of paramount importance here, and providing mouth care or giving a small piece of fruit before meals may, alongside the aroma of food, stimulate the appetite (unless there is a food aversion).

The aesthetics of eating in a clean, relaxed environment, being painfree, unhurried and in a quiet atmosphere are important. It has

Table 2. Why does the taste change?

Suggestions	Cause	Source
Tumour by product	Amino acids produced by the tumour lower the threshold for other bitter stimuli	de Wyss and Walteresk (1975)
Reduced rate of cell turnover	A response of the whole system to cancer	de Wyss and Walteresk (1975)
Trace metals altered, e.g. zinc	Tumour or drugs	Henkin and Schecter (1976)
Poor oral hygiene	Saliva reduced Tongue coated Bacterial byproducts Infections	Twycross and Lack (1986)
Radiotherapy, oral surgery	Mucositis and decreased saturation	Strohl (1983)
Food aversion	Related to previous treatment	Bernstein and Bernstein (1981)

Taste change	Nursing intervention Coping strategy
Higher threshold for sweetness	Add seasoning
Lower threshold urea (meat tastes bad)	Avoid meat and vegetable protein
Coffee and chocolate	Avoid

been suggested that sometimes the 'meat aversion factor' in cancer patients increases through the day so advantage can be taken of this by providing a high-protein breakfast (Strohl, 1983) or looking at alternative sources of protein.

The differences for the terminally ill do need to be further investigated. The philosophy for the oncology patient may be to treat food as a sort of 'medicine' to be taken — this certainly is not the case in the terminally ill. Similarly, zinc therapy would be viewed with caution due to side-effects. However, some drugs already in use may be helping the problem, e.g. haloperidol, and successful strategies using hypnosis have been reported (Strohl, 1983).

The Dehydration Question

One important question relates to a reduced fluid intake as the terminally ill patient approaches death. Providing nourishment is symbolically very important to the patient, family and health care team. It has been observed that the symptoms associated with dehydration seem to be much milder in the terminally ill, i.e. mostly those of thirst and a dry mouth (Anon, 1986).

Using intravenous fluids at this stage has been seriously questioned, with Oliver demonstrating that blood chemistry can be maintained to near normal, apart from a raised urea, without i.v. fluids (Oliver, 1984). Meanwhile, Dolan (1983) and Zerwekh (1983) suggest the detrimental effects of intravenous fluids, including increased flow of urine, production of gastrointestinal fluids and secretions. The fluids may in fact cause an exacerbation of ascites or increase oedema around the tumour. Dolan has observed two groups of patients where renal shutdown in both had been recognized as an important indication of approaching death. The group receiving i.v. therapy required oropharyngeal suction and their death was not described as 'comfortable'. Nursing intervention will be aimed at providing good mouth care, as for a dry mouth (see previous section), appropriate symptom management, e.g. associated nausea and restlessness, and sensitive teaching of both the patient and family related to the agreed management of the dehydrating patient.

Nausea and Vomiting

Nausea will obviously have an impact on dietary intake and like pain is difficult to quantify and describe, relying on measures of subjective distress (Rhodes, Watson and Johnson, 1984). In the authors' experience many patients say that they prefer to vomit intermittently than to have the continuous problem of nausea. Certainly antiemetics seem to control the vomiting more quickly than the nausea.

Both these problems will have an impact on the electrolyte balance, hydration and nutritional status of the patient and hence an impact on other concurrent symptoms, often linked with the need to change the route of drug administration. It is interesting that much of the focus for managing these problems has been researched in the oncology patient receiving cytotoxic therapy. In a sense this seems to have mimicked the development of strategies regarding pain, i.e. reviewing antiemetic drug therapy, devising methods to assess the problem (Rhodes, Watson and Johnson, 1984), adjustments in local factors that can affect nausea and vomiting (Flaharty, 1985), and the development of behavioural techniques to help the patient influence his own subjective experience (Twycross and Lack, 1987).

For the patient with advanced cancer admitted to Michael Sobell House, Oxford, Twycross and Lack estimate that the problem affects more than 40 per cent of their patients.

Using animal and human studies, the reflex pathways involved in vomiting have been described with the impact of morphine on these pathways (Bindeman, Milsted, Kaye, Welsh, Habeshaw, Calman).

The chemoreceptor trigger zone (CTZ) is a small area of the brain stimulated by specific *drugs, chemicals*, and by products of cells. The vomiting centre can also be triggered by the cerebral cortex, i.e. sight, smell and psychological factors. 'Motion sickness' occurs when impulses travel from the vestibular area to the vomiting centre via the cerebellum and the other major mechanism involves the abdominal viscera, e.g. the 'squashed stomach syndrome' (Twycross and Lack, 1986), constipation. Assessment and management of nausea and vomiting needs continued observation to isolate the cause and the combination of antiemetics that may be required (Flaharty, 1985; Twycross and Lack, 1986). (See Figure 3.)

Management will also require appropriate use of alternative methods of drug administration, e.g. at Strathcarron Hospice the use of the syringe driver. Antiemetics can be combined with other medication, thus relieving the patient of further gastrointestinal disturbance (Allwood, 1984; Badger and Regnard, 1986).

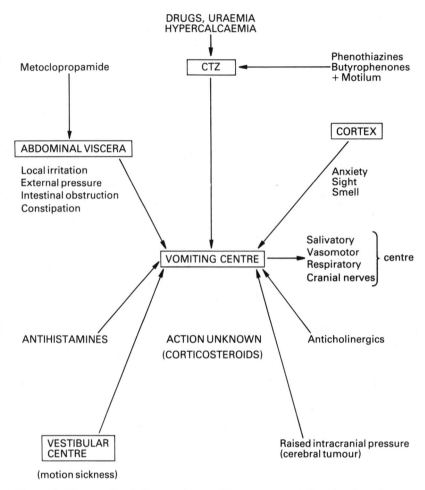

Figure 3. Factors that influence the vomiting centre and site of action of some of the common antiemetic drugs (adapted from Twycross and Lack (1986)

Dietary Measures

As well as advice regarding the use of drug therapy, dietary adjustments can be made — these can be related to the effects that certain foods have. Certainly a useful area for investigation would include what food, odour, temperature and mixture of food should be avoided (Flaharty, 1985; Stuart and Duffy, 1986).

If trends of the oncology specialist are to be followed, then assessing the role of anxiety in this area should be included. The authors also believe that behavioural techniques, guided imagery and relaxation may be of great value as an adjunct to drug therapy (Bindeman *et al.*, 1981).

Impaired Sleep

A search reveals no specific qualitative research related to sleep in the terminally ill, whether managed within hospital, home or a hospice environment. One patient in Strathcarron woke recently asking repeatedly for reassurance that nothing would happen to him; he then admitted his real fear — death. Of those patients referred to Strathcarron, 24 per cent complained of insomnia. Much has been written about sleep within the hospital environment (Wilson-Barnett, 1978; Bailey, 1981; Carter, 1985) and for two patients in Hockley's study sleepless nights continued for three and four nights before death (Hockley, 1983). Hartman (1970) believes that adequate sleep supplies the patient with a feeling of being rested and will also be able to enhance both physical and mental functioning (Carter, 1985). Carter further suggests that qualitative as well as quantitative measurement needs to be made.

Lamb (1982) has compared sleeping patterns of patients with malignant and non-malignant diseases and concluded that oncology patients did not seem to have different sleep patterns. This was despite their relatively higher level of anxiety and depression as measured. However, this study may have had some design weakness.

Assessment involves many factors:

Focal, e.g.
   Pain
   Nausea
   Anxiety
Contextual, e.g.
   Noise
   Temperature
   Light

The importance of assisting with this problem is that it will have an impact not only on the patient but, if at home, then also on his family.

Suggestions

Certainly management with short-acting hypnotics can quickly alleviate insomnia but other areas of interest include incidence of dreams and nightmares. It would also be useful to look at the overall activity of the patient and at other nursing strategies that can help induce sleep in the terminally ill. Interventions planned to alleviate other problems may also obviously reduce sleep disturbance.

Oedema

Oedema was a problem for 50 per cent of patients in Hockley's study and can be defined as 'excess asccumulation of fluid in the interstitial component of the extracellular fluid compartment' (Swedborg, 1984). In these patients lymphoedema, cerebral oedema and ascites may produce the most distress.

Lymphoedema

Alteration of the normal lymphatic channels as a result of surgery (e.g. mastectomy), tumour involvement or radiotherapy can be seen as swollen upper or lower limbs in the terminally ill. Not only causing physical discomfort affecting mobility or body image, lymphoedema may be complicated by cellulitis and lymphangitis (Swedborg, 1984). Figure 4 presents influencing factors in the development of lymphoedema.

Currently, intervention involves elevation, the use of elastic sleeves/ stockings, exercises, massage and pneumatic compression, e.g. using a Jobst pump. It has been demonstrated that graded elastic compression stockings with 24 mmHg pressure at the ankle are effective in decreasing size of symptoms when used over a one-week period (McNair, Martin and Orr, 1976). Similarly with upper limbs reduction in volume of oedema can be achieved using elastic sleeve in conjunction with pneumatic compression.

Assessment of the extent of the lymphoedema and prevention of complication are essential in the early stages. New developments are shared as the British Lymphology Group is established. More sophisticated (and more comfortable) compression pumps are becoming available, e.g. the ten-chambered sequential model.

It will be interesting to review studies evaluating the different regimens of care, and certainly nursing interventions will include teaching new skills to both patient and family.

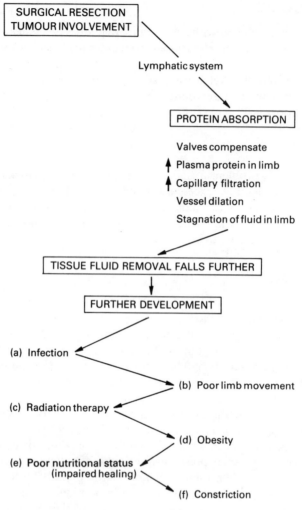

Figure 4. Development of lymphoedema

Impaired Wound Healing

Any type of tissue breakdown in terminal disease can prove to be intensely distressing, not only because of the physical discomfort it causes but also because of the related psychological effects (Wells, 1984). 'It just doesn't belong to me', said one patient as she gazed at a huge cavity in her abdominal wall, — 'and anyway, how can you hug your grandchildren with *that*?' Much has been written about wound healing and tissue viability (Westaby, 1983; Torrance, 1984; Barton and Barton, 1981) and there are a vast array of new products to assist in this process. The challenge of solving the very varied wound problems in terminal disease is not only caught up with the nature of the wound itself — we also need to know and be able to assess the range of predisposing factors. In this framework can be included 'internal' lesions, e.g. fistulas as well as fungating breast lesions and decubitus ulcers.

Some Influencing Factors (after Roy)

Contextual factors, e.g.

> Stress
> Other pathology
> Nutritional status
> Drug therapy, e.g. N.S.A.I.

Focal factors, e.g.

> Unsatisfactory wound environment

Residual factors, e.g.

> Age
> Poor circulation

Boore (1979) has already demonstrated the impact of stress on wound healing in postoperative patients — the situation would be interesting to review relative to wound status in the terminally ill. Nutritional status has its impact on materials available for repair — proteins, carbohydrates, fats, vitamins and minerals (zinc and iron) (Table 3).

Drugs to be considered include the effect of steroids and non-steroidal anti-inflammatory agents on healing as well as the direct effects of cytotoxic therapy and the subtle influences of opiates on patients' spontaneous movement in response to pressure (Torrance, 1983).

Nursing interventions should be based on maintaining an ideal wound environment. Temperature should be kept constant to encourage white

Table 3. Nutritional status and wound healing. Adapted from Carrieri,
            Lindsey and West (1986)

The problem	The effect
Poor protein intake	Poor revascularization Collagen synthesis Fibroblast production
Poor carbohydrate intake	Protein breakdown
Undernutrition leads to deficiencies in linoleic acids	Poor cell membrane and prostaglandin production
Reduced vitamin C	Reduced vessel production, collagen synthesis and antibacterial substance (superoxide)
Reduced vitamin B	No marked effect
Reduced vitamin A	Epithelialization (may use Vit. A in *chronic* steroid users to counteract anti-inflammatory action)
Reduced Vitamin K	Impact on coagulation and bleeding
Minerals (zinc):	Enzyme action impaired.
Reduced zinc	Healing not necessarily improved by zinc supplements if normal serum zinc

cell activity and mitotic activity and dressing changes should be rapid
and wounds only cleansed when really necessary. The acid-base balance
should also be maintained by using comparable lotions to ensure good
cell mobility and phagocytosis. Oxygen is essential for cellular activity
and can only be ensured by good circulation to the wound and oxygen-
permeable dressings. (Directing pure oxygen on to the wound does
not increase the available oxygen for cellular activity.) Moisture is
essential for all wound healing and, of course, movement of wound
edges and infection should also be avoided. All these principles are
based on work by Torrance (1984) and Barton and Barton (1981).

So the patient needs an odour-free, comfortable dressing that
enhances self-image and disturbs him as little as possible. He also
needs to feel involved in the planning of the management and the
change of the wound even if progress is not being made.

The health care team need to be able to provide continuity of care.
Subjective assessments can often be much helped by simple devices to
trace size and shape of wounds on polythene even if a 3D picture is
not so easy to obtain. (The use of silastic foam has helped greatly in
comparing wound size changes.)

For the wound the environment needs to be moist, nutrient-rich with little wound interference. Barton's philosophy of never putting into a granulating wound what you wouldn't put into your own eye does reinforce the delicate balance in the environment of granulating tissue. Eusol is nephrotoxic and Aserbine delays healing response (Barton and Barton, 1981).

Special Problems — Realistic Goals

Literature on the problems of the terminally ill can be subsumed under the following headings:

1. Ulcerating metastatic lesions
2. Pressure sores
3. Fistulas

The first of these, Ulcerating metastatic lesions, seems most pertinent and specifically relevant to this book. Here the wound has developed from extension of tumour into the epithelium and is associated with capillary rupture, necrosis and infection.

These lesions are most commonly associated with breast cancer but also occur with cancers of head and neck, lung, uterus, kidney, ovary and colon, as well as melanoma and lymphoma. Where the problem cannot be removed (e.g. by surgery or radiotherapy), then the realistic goals as stated by Foltz (1980) are minimizing infection, bleeding and odour.

It is interesting to compare the principles of management of Foltz (1980) and Sims and Fitzgerald (1985).

Cleansing

Both suggest showering or bathing and the value of the nurses' ungloved hand to enable the patient to view the wound with less disgust. However, the scrubbing action and use of detergents which break surface fat would seem particularly non-selective in the type of tissue being removed (Foltz, 1980).

Wound debridement

Deeper lesions, both studies suggest, may warrant surgical debridement, but obviously the patient's condition may be such that debridement may not be a realistic goal. The authors have made a silastic foam 'breastplate' — used for the last days of a lady with a necrotic lesion. The main aim here was comfort and a pain-free dressing. Agents differ, but the emphasis has changed from 'reducing the burning sensation by reducing the concentration of the debriding solution used!' to a more sensitive approach to the needs of the wound — the use of viscopaste PB7, varidase (valuable when the area is not vascular as it is harmless to healthy tissue) in conjunction with barrier cream and confeel. Icing sugar acts to debride and deodorize (Sims and Fitzgerald, 1985) but is painful if in contact with healthy tissue.

It is interesting that despite the harm that gauze swabs can do to wounds when granulation is the goal (Sims and Fitzgerald, 1985) it may be they have a place in debridement (Neuberger, 1987).

Haemostasis

Dressing design and removal play an important part in capillary bleeding. The 'dried-out gauze swab' being everything a wound does not need, prevention (the moist wound environment) is best but otherwise soaking off with warm normal saline or hydrogen peroxide (5 volume solution) mixed with 2 per cent xylocaine. Ice and pressure are often inappropriate but caustic pencil, adrenoline 1–1000 and oxycel are recommended by Sims and Fitzgerald (1985).

Reducing infection/odour control

The wound swab may reveal anaerobic organisms, and malodorous lesions have been much helped by metronidazole (Flagyl) (Jones, Willis and Ferguson, 1978; Sparrow, Hinton and Rubes, 1980; Ashford et al., 1984) topically or systemically. Live yoghurt also has a value in odour control. David (1985) reported on a small study using special Lyofoam C dressings which moulded well on difficult shapes but Draper reports 'lateral strikethrough' as a disadvantage.

Povidone iodine (10 per cent) and liquid paraffin (50/50) has bacterostatic properties and recently there have been changes in its presentation (inadine). Obviously sensitivity to iodine would preclude its use, and it can accumulate systemically and cause renal failure (Barton and Barton, 1981). It is also not very good for body image, often staining garments.

Foltz (1980), Draper (1985) and Sims and Fitzgerald (1985) have compared the lotions and dressings available with comments related to their use. The challenge lies in using current research to the best advantage of the patient. Do we need to meet all the criteria for the ideal wound environment even if total healing is not a realistic goal? Do these principles support the comfort needs of the patient?

Future research may need to look more closely at the psychosocial aspects of coping with wounds and the impact on quality of life, moving forward towards a more accurate assessment and evaluation both subjectively and objectively.

Impaired Elimination

Another problem is constipation — described as infrequent, irregular passage of hard faeces with associated difficulty and occasional pain. This is not an uncommon problem in terminal disease and if ignored leads to even greater distress, as the person feels lethargic, has a thick-coated tongue, may feel nauseated, vomit or have little or no appetite. Forty-one per cent of patients referred to Strathcarron Hospice were identified as being constipated. Historically, nursing management of this problem in the adult population in hospital has relied heavily on the use of enemata, suppositories and laxatives (Royal Marsden Hospital, 1984). Reviewing the causes and planning individual care have been increasingly the aims of care.

Why is Constipation such a Problem in the Terminally Ill?

It is easy to link factors that will predispose the terminally ill patient to constipation. An altered dietary intake associated with anorexia or dysphagia will have a direct effect on the constituents and mass of the stool. The patient who is poorly hydrated or whose pattern of mobility is compromised due to lymphoedema, paraplegia or general weakness, and the patient who is experiencing psychological changes, e.g. depression, will be at risk. Similarly, the patient whose tumour is causing a mechanical obstruction of the gastrointestinal tract or whose medication is affecting gut mortility, the patient who is experiencing local discomfort due to haemorrhoids or fissures, and the patient whose environment does not enable easy access to facilities and essential privacy, will all require careful assessment.

Many terminally ill patients are unable to gain access to a toilet independently and many have little enough strength to maintain the posture or perform the action. Bedpans require the patient to use 50 per cent more oxygen than a commode (Lewind, 1972) and commodes can be uncomfortable and lacking in dignity if thought is not given to siting in the ward or the home. Many patients lack their own 'sacral padding' although special covered foam seats can be obtained to ease this problem.

Twycross and Lack (1986, pp. 166–207) quote the seven litres of secretion that pour into the system daily, and we only need to think of the shedding of cells and tissues, yet for some patients the logic may be, 'I'm not eating — so I don't need a bowel movement'.

Constipation is not defined in quantitative ways because it is not possible to describe what is physiologically normal in numerical terms (Godding, 1980). Thus the variation from person to person must be assessed in terms of size, consistency and ease of passage as well as frequency (Cimprich, 1985).

Anticipatory care can alleviate much distress and one of the areas where it is easy to anticipate problems is related to opiate therapy. Eighty to ninety per cent of patients receiving morphine become constipated. Reduced mobility of the bowel is associated also with increased electrolyte and water absorption as well as sphincter effects (Twycross and Lack, 1986). It is known that the larger the dose used the greater the likelihood of reduced function; also, chronic narcotic use often results in a chronic bowel problem, as cited by Cimprich (1985).

Because many of the problems that predispose the terminally ill patient to constipation are a direct result of either their pathology, its effects or the treatment, goals must be realistic. High-fibre diets are often not an option in very advanced disease and neither will be withdrawal of analgesic.

'Treat the patient not the constipation' (Aman, 1980) will often produce results as concomitant distressing symptoms are treated. It is useful to remember that in addition to the foods we naturally associate with a high-fibre content, cereals, root vegetables and fruit, older, more natural fruits and vegetables do produce a greater laxative effect. If patients require foods that are softer, Cimprich (1985) uses the following sources of fibre:

Bananas
Apple sauce
Cooked vegetables
Peanut butter
Cocoa
Chocolate (coffee)

The following agents are relevant:
Faecal softeners
Osmotic laxatives
Per rectum evacuants
Bulk-forming agents
Contact cathartics

Faecal softeners, e.g. dioctyl sodium sulphosuccinate (Dioctyl) surface wetting agent. This enhances absorption of water and increases faecal water content. Dose: up to 500 mg divided.

Osmotic laxatives. These are sugars, e.g. lactulose or magnesium salts (e.g. magnesium hydroxide). Because these substances are not absorbed or poorly absorbed, fluid is retained in the bowel lumen, softening the stool and stimulating contraction of the colon.

Bulk-forming agents, e.g. bran methyl cellulose mucilloids (Fybogel, Regulan). By retaining water in the stool, they increase stool bulk and stimulate peristalsis. Obviously not of use in contraindicated faecal impaction, they are safe but large quantities of bran are required to achieve a response.

Contact laxatives. These stimulate intestinal peristalsis and cause H_2O (water) and electrolyte secretion (see Table 4).

For patients on opiate therapy each patient profile includes those factors that predispose to constipation (see p. 109), as well as a record of bowel function — size, consistency, frequency and associated intervention. It is customary in the absence of a bowel action to perform a rectal examination every three days — this may in fact seem ironic where 'individual patient care' is the shared aim.

Regimens are based on experience of the problems and often include a combination of systemic drugs titrated to achieve a bowel motion that is comfortable for the patient. For the terminally ill the long-term effect of laxative therapy can be effectively ignored, yet it would be of value to review the ease which some of these medications can be taken (tablet, number of tablets).

Pirrie (1980) suggests that manual evacuation is too painful and dangerous and should be performed by medical staff. Enemata can be very useful in softening impacted faeces, e.g. arachis oil enema, or evacuating the rectum as a result of mucosal stimulation, e.g. phosphate enema. However, the hazards of soap solutions and tap water must remove these from the options (Smith, 1967; Lewin, 1976).

The nursing role should involve information and teaching about the effect of narcotic drugs and how the patient can help in observation

Table 4. Action of contact laxatives

Name	Action	Comments
e.g. Bisacodyl tablets	Mainly act on large bowel. Can lead to an atonic colon	Can cause abdominal cramps. Long-term use
Sodium picosulphate (Picolax)	Acts within 10–14 hr	Usually taken at night
Danthron (Dorbanex) (mix with warm H_2O) (capsules)	Mainly large bowel	No longer available
Senna (tablets × 4 tabs)	Large bowel only	May colour urine red

of his stool. Cimprich states that studies have demonstrated that senokot (anthraqurine derivative) does reverse narcotic-induced constipation (Cimprich, 1985).

It would be interesting to review more closely the true incidence of constipation in terminal disease and compare the effectiveness of different regimes. Management and assessment seem to be fundamental here and the development of a systemic approach would be of value.

Fatigue

One of the symptoms not identified by Hockley but found distressing is fatigue. This in fact has been identified in a study of 30 cancer patients receiving radiotherapy (Haylock and Hart, 1979) and in a study of newly diagnosed lung cancer patients (McCorkle, Benoliel and Donaldson, 1979) and is often cited in the terminally ill. Piper (1986) cites the absence of an 'interdisciplinary definition of fatigue' and also reports that fatigue can be recoverable by rest where others believe it is caused by rest and lessened by exercise.

The question arises — is fatigue a particular problem for the terminally ill? Certainly where acute fatigue may be likened to acute pain, i.e. serving a protective function, chronic fatigue serves no purpose and can interfere with many activities that could enhance quality of life. Piper cites several factors that may be associated with fatigue. Currently intervention related to alleviating this symptom involves the employment of further drug therapy in the form of steroids. However, there may be many implications and challenges to review nursing practices relating to this concept.

Conclusion

The nature of the preceding section may have highlighted the problem as we attempt to outline the nature of nursing management of the terminally ill patient and his family. Patient-centred care involves a sensitivity to their special needs, yet in order to be credible our 'expertise' needs to be evaluated.

Hospice care can be a rather elite area managing a specific disease model, yet the future must look at the implications of these principles in other settings, i.e. with other diseases and in other environments. It may be that hospices have an ideal opportunity both in terms of work environment (Mills and Pennoni, 1986) and patient populaton to tackle the problems of nursing research in terminal care, despite the 'newness' of this and the lack of prepared nurse researchers (Petrosino, 1986).

References

Ahman, R.A. (1980) Treating the patient not the constipation, *American Journal of Nursing*, **80**, 1634–1635.

Allwood, M.C. (1984) Diamorphine mixed with anti-emetic drugs in plastic syringes, *British Journal of Pharmaceutical Practice*, **6**, 131, 88–90.

Anon (1986) Terminal dehydration, *Lancet*, **i**, 306.

Ashford, R., Plat, G., Maner, J., and Teare, L. (1984) Double blind trial of metronidazole in malodorous ulcerating tumours, Letter, *Lancet*, **i**, 1232.

Badger, C., and Regnard, C. (1986) Pumping in pain relief, *Nursing Times*, **82** (28), 52–54.

Bailey, H. (1981) *Sleep and the Hospital Patient*. Department of Nursing and Community Health Studies, The Polytechnic of the South Bank Research Report 1.

Barton, A.A., and Barton, M. (1981) *The Management and Prevention of Pressure Sores*. Faber & Faber, London.

Bernstein, I., and Bernstein, I.D. (1981) Learned food aversions and cancer anorexia. *Cancer Treatment Report*, **65**, (Suppl. 5), 43–47.

Bersani, G., and Carl, W. (1983) Oral care for cancer patients, *American Journal of Nursing*, **4**, 533–536.

Bindeman, S., Calman, K.C., Milsted, R.A.V., and Trotter, J.M. (1981) Enhancement of quality of life with relaxation training in cancer patients attending a chemotherapy unit. In Watson, M., and Greer, S. (eds) *Psychosocial Issues in Malignant Disease*. Proceedings of the First Annual Conference of the British Psychosocial Oncology Group, London, 7–8 Nov. Pergamon Press, Oxford.

Boore, J. (1979) *Fit For Recovery*. RCN Publications, London.

Bruno, P. (1979) The nature of wound healing — implication for nursing practice, *Nurs. Clin. North America*, **14**, 4.

Carrieri, V., Lindsey, A. M., and West, C. (1986). *Pathophysiological Phenomena in Jursing*. W. A. Saunders, Philadelphia.

Carter, D. (1985) In need of a good night's sleep, *Nursing Times*, **81** (46), 24–26.

Cheater, F. (1985) Xerostomia in malignant disease. Clinical Revision Series. II, *Nursing Mirror*, **161** (3), 177.

Cimprich, B. (1985) *Cancer Nursing Supplement* 1, 39–43.

Corr, A., and Corr, M. (1983) *Hospice Care Principles and Practice*. Springer, New York.

Daeffler, R.J. (1986) Oral care. *Hospice Journal*, **2** (1), 81–102.

David, J. (1985) Dressing fungating wounds, *Nursing Mirror*, **161** (16), 27–28.

de Wyss, W.D., and Walters, K. (1975) Abnormalities of taste sensation in cancer.

Dolan, M. (1983) Another hospice nurse says, *Nursing*, **83**, 51.

Draper, J. (1985) Make the dressing fit the wound, *Nursing Times*, **81** (41), 32–35.

Flaharty, A.M. (1985) Symptom management: Nausea and vomiting, *Cancer Nursing*, **8**, 36–38.

Foltz, A.T. (1980) Nursing care of ulcerating metastatic lesions, *Oncology Nursing Forum*, **7**, No. 2.

Godding, E.W. (1976) Therapeutics of laxative agents with special reference to the anthraquinones, *Pharmacology*, **14** (Suppl.), 78–101.

Godding, E.W. (1980) Investigating constipation, *British medical Journal*, **280**, 15–38.

Grobe, M., Ilstrup, D., and Ahman, D. (1981) Skills needed by family members to maintain the care of an advanced cancer patient; *Cancer Nursing*, October, 371–375.

Hallett, N. (1984) Mouth care, *Nursing Mirror*, **159** (21), 31–33.

Hartman, E.L. (1970) What is good sleep? *International Psychiatry Clinics*, **7**, 59–69.

Hawkett, S. (1986) Educational opportunities in terminal care, Hospice Manager Forum, RCN Paper 30, October.

Haylock, P.J. Hart, L.K. and McCorkle, R. (1979) Fatigue in patients receiving local radiation, *Cancer Nursing*, **2**, 461–467.

Henkin, R.I., and Schecter, P.J. (1976) A double blind study on the effects of zinc sulphate on taste and smell distinction, *American Journal of Medical Science*, **272**, 285–299.

Hockley, J. (1983) An investigation to identify symptoms of distress in the terminally ill patient and his/her family in the general medical ward. Unpublished research report.

Holland, J., Rowland, J., and Plumb, M. (1977) Psychological aspects of anorexia in cancer patients, *Cancer Research*, **37**, 2425–2428.

Holmes, S., and Dickerson, J. (1987) The quality of life design and evaluation of a self assessment instrument for use with cancer patients, *International Journal of Nursing Studies*, **24** (1), 15–23.

Jaffe, J., and Martin, W.R. (1980) Opioid analgesics and antagonistics. In Gilman, A. *et al.* (eds) *Pharmacological Basis of Therapeutics*, 6th edn. Macmillan, New York, pp. 494–534.

Jones, P., Willis, A., and Ferguson, I. (1978) Treatment of anaerobically infected pressure sores with topical metastatic breast cancer, *American Journal of Nursing*, **73** (6), 1034.

Kershaw, B., and Salvage, J. (1986) *Models for Nursing*, Wiley, Chichester.

Lamb, M. (1982) Sleeping patterns of patients with malignant and non-malignant diseases, *Cancer Nursing*, October, 389.

Lane, B., and Forgay, W. (1981) Updating your oral hygiene protocol for the patient with cancer, *Canadian Nurse*, **77**, 22–29.

Lant, A. (ed.) (1986) Gastrointestinal system 19. Constipation, *Mims Magazine*, Oct. 1, ii.

Lewin, D. (1976) Care of the constipated patient, *Nursing Times*, **72**, 444–446.

MacCaughey, A.M. (1968) *A Comprehensive Physical Therapy Programme for the Post Mastectomy Lymphedema Patient*. American Physical Therapy Association.

Manning, M. (1984) *The Hospice Alternative*. Souvenir Press, London.

McCorkle, Benoliel, and Donaldson, G. (1979–81) *A Manual of Data Collection Instruments*. Seattle University of Washington, Community Health Care Systems, 1979–81.

McNair, T.J., Martin, I.J., and Orr, J.D. (1976) Intermittent compression for lymphedema of arm, *Clinical Onocology*, **2**, 339–342.

McCorkle, R., and Young, K. (1978) Development of a symptom distress scale. *Cancer Nurisng*, **1**, 373–378.

Mills, D., and Pennoni, M. (1986) A nurturing work environment, *Cancer Nursing*, **9** (3), 17–24.

Mills, W.D. (1983) Care of the dying in hospital. Unpublished MSC thesis, University of Glasgow.

Mumford, S.P. (1984) Can high fibre diets improve bowel function in patients on a radiotherapy ward? Unpublished project for the English Board Course on Care of the Dying, Oxford.

Neuberger, G. (1987) Wound care, *Nursing*, **17** (2), 34–37.

Oliver, D.J. (1984) Terminal dehydration, *Lancet*, **11**, 631.

Petrosino, B. (1986) Research challenges in hospice nursing, *The Hospice Journal*, **2** (1), 1–10.

Pierson, S., Pierson, D., Swallow, R., and Johnson, G. (1983) Efficacy of graded elastic compression in the lower leg, *JMA*, **249** (2), 242.

Piper, B.F. (1986) Fatigue. In Carrieri, V., Lindsey, A.M., and West, C., *Pathophysiological Phenomena in Nursing*. W.B. Saunders, Philadelphia.

Pirrie, J. (1980) Constipation in the elderly. *Nursing* (1st series), **17**, 753–754.

Ranier, J.K., O'Donnell, T.T., Kalisher, L., and Darling, R.C. (1977) Selection of patients with lymphedema for compression therapy, *The American Journal of Surgery*, **133**, 430–438.

Rhodes, V., Watson, P., and Johnson, M. (1984) Development of reliable and valid measures of nausea and vomiting, *Cancer Nursing*, **1**, 34–41.

Riehl, J., and Roy, C. (eds) (1980) *Conceptual Models for Nursing Practice*. Appleton-Century-Crofts, Norwich, CT.

Royal Marsden Hospital (1984) *Manual of Clinical Nursing Policies and Procedures*. Harper & Row, London.

Schnipper, I.M. (1985) Symptom management. Anorexia. *Cancer Nursing*, Suppl. 1.

Sims, S. (1986) Slow stroke back massage for cancer patients, *Nursing Times*, **82** (13), 47–50.

Sims, R., and Fitzgerald, V. (1985) Community nursing management of patients with ulcerating/fungating malignant breast disease. RCN publication.

Smith, D. (1967) Severe anaphylactic reaction after soap enema, *British Medical Journal*, **214** (4), 215.

Sparrow, G., Minton, M., and Rubes, R. (1980) Metronidazole in smelly tumours, Letter to the editor, *Lancet*, **1**, 1185.

Strohl, R.A. (1983) Nursing management of the patient with cancer experiencing taste changes, *Cancer Nursing*, **6** (5), 353–359.

Stuart, E., and Duffy, J. (1986) *We Can Help*. Dietary booklet, Oncology Department, Gartnavel General Hospital, Glasgow.

Swedborg, Iwona (1984) Effects of treatment with an elastic sleeve and intermittent pneumatic compression in post mastectomy patients with lymphedema of the arm, *Scand. J. Rehabb.*, **16**, 35–41.

Torrance, C., (1983) *Pressure Sores, Aetiology, Treatment and Prevention*. Croom Helm, London.

Twycross, R., and Lack, S. (1986) *Control of Alimentary Symptoms in Far Advanced Cancer*. Churchill Livingstone, Edinburgh.

Wells, R. (1984) Wound care, *Nursing Mirror*, **158** (10), 10–15.

Westerby, S. (ed.) (1985) *Wound Care*. Heinemann, London.

White, M.B. (1972) Importance of selected nursing activities, *Nursing Research*, **21** (1), 4–14.

Wilson-Barnett, J. (1978) In hospital: Patients' feelings and opinions, *Nursing Times* Occasional Paper 78, **74** (11), 29–34.

Zerwekh, J.V. (1983) The dehydration question, *Nursing*, **83**, 47–51.

Part 5 Comfort Care

Nursing Issues and Research in Terminal Care
Edited by J. Wilson-Barnett and J. Raiman
© 1988 John Wiley & Sons Ltd.

CHAPTER 7

Pain and its Management

JENNIFER RAIMAN

'Illness is the doctor to whom we pay most heed; to kindness, to
knowledge we make promises only, pain we obey.'

Marcel Proust (1871–1922)

Introduction

Pain in dying patients whilst not inevitable may be present and in all
but a few patients can be relieved, e.g. 50 per cent of patients with
advanced cancer may have no pain or only minor discomfort. However,
the rest too often fail to get the relief that could be provided — though
the control of pain is the key to all other care.

Whilst death may occur suddenly, often there is a protracted period
of time during which it is evident that no radical cure will be possible.
Then the emphasis of approach shifts from the insular mental state of
'pathological process and disease orientation' and is centred upon
understanding and reacting to the needs of the whole person. The test
for therapeutic success is: 'How well are the symptoms being relieved?'

Concentration alone on the role of professional knowledge and
technical excellence without patient participation ignores and devalues
the 'whole person' dimension in suffering. If pain is perceived in
isolation as a separate entity, the potential for suffering in dying
patients is increased and the opportunities for greater understanding
and relief decreased and lost.

Good pain control requires both *sensitivity* to the patient's needs on
every level and the *competence* to meet them.

Limitations

To cover the topic of pain fully is beyond the scope of this chapter. I
have tried therefore to outline with a 'broad brush' some of the

dimensions of pain and to indicate current understanding, practice and developments for its assessment and relief.

I hope this approach and framework will stimulate further thought and reading, and enhance the concept of patient participation and individualized care.

Neurophysiological Pain Theories

Historically pain has been a subject for debate and enquiry over the centuries.

Present understanding on the nature of pain has been formulated and dominated by three major theoretical concepts:

1. Specificity
2. Pattern
3. Gate control theory

which when linked to the action of the recently identified morphine-like substances endorphins and enkephalins enables the experience of pain to be viewed as a merger of neurophysiological and psychological components:

1. Sensory/perceptual
2. Emotional/motivational
3. Cognitive/evaluative.

The Specificity Theory

The specificity theory originated from Descartes' observation in 1644 of a 'straight through' concept from the skin to the brain, assuming that pain receptors existed in the brain, forming a pain centre. Descartes proposed that the system is like the bell-ringing mechanism in a church: a man pulls the rope at the bottom of the tower and the bell rings in the belfry. Thus the stimulus of pain 'sets particles into activity and the motion is transmitted through the body into the head where an alarm system is set off'.

The theory underwent little change until the nineteenth century, when Johannes Muller in 1838 set out a series of propositions relating to the 'specific energies' and 'specific irritability' of the nerves. In addition, Muller described four major cutaneous modalities, touch, warmth, cold and pain. Von Frey between 1894 and 1895 linked together and expanded upon the cutaneous modality concept, presuming each to have its own special projected system to the brain where it was appropriately interpreted. Secondly he considered that the specialization of end organs was anatomical and gave each of the few established modalities to one of the end organs. Thus the free nerve endings were for pain. Krause end bulbs for cold, Ruffini endings for warmth, and touch was given to the Meissner corpuscles round the hair follicles and in the skin. He postulated that since free nerve endings were to be found almost everywhere as were pain spots, the free nerve endings were pain receptors.

Although the specificity theory has formed the basis for much of the research into pain, particularly in the first half of this century, physiological and psychological evidence gradually accumulated to refute or extend its conclusions.

There is physiological evidence that specialization exists within the sensory system. There is none to show that stimulation of one type of receptor fibre or spinal pathway elicits sensations of only a single psychological modality such as pain (Melzack and Wall, 1982).

The Pattern Theory

A number of theories have been proposed which can be grouped together under the general heading of 'pattern theory'. Goldscheider (1898) suggested that stimulus intensity and central summation are the critical determinants of pain. According to this concept, pain results when the total output of the cells exceeds a critical level.

The simplest form of pattern theory deals primarily with peripheral rather than central patterning, i.e. pain is considered to be due to excessive peripheral stimulation that produces a pattern of nerve impulses which is interpreted centrally as pain.

Livingston (1943) was the first to suggest pain-specific central neural mechanisms. He proposed that pathological stimulation of sensory nerves initiated activity in reverberating circuits (closed, self-exciting loops of neurons) in the grey matter of the spinal cord (cited by Melzack and Wall, 1982).

The Gate Theory

In 1965 Melzack and Wall published a model for the dorsal horn circuitry responsible for pain transmission. They called the model the 'gate control system'. The starting point for the gate theory was their belief that neither the specificity theory (that pain has its own peripheral and central apparatus) nor the pattern theory (that pain results from intense stimulation of non-specific receptors) could account for what is known as pain.

Melzack and Wall made a specific proposal concerning the organization of a spinal cord 'gating mechanism'. The theory of 1965 proposed that a mechanism in the dorsal horns of the spinal cord acts like a gate which can increase or decrease the flow of nerve impulses from peripheral fibres to the central nervous system. When the amount of information that passes through the gate exceeds a critical level, it activates the neural area responsible for pain experience and response.

The existence of a *central control trigger* was suggested as the mechanism that activated the higher processes such as anxiety, anticipation, attention and past experience, all of which have a powerful influence on the experience of pain and exert control over the sensory input.

The impact of the gate theory has been considerable in both clinical and research fields. In 1978 Wall published a reexamination and restatement of the theory in the light of new evidence. He emphasized the complex nature of the excitatory–inhibitory organization of the transmitting cells of the substantia gelatinosa, although the mechanism of inhibition remains as yet unknown.

Whilst debate and controversy continue, the original concept of a 'gating mechanism' has the capacity (singularly unachieved before) to clarify and link together the complex physiological, anatomical and psychological phenomena of pain.

The proposed existence of a 'gating mechanism' resulted in the development and use of dorsal column stimulation (DCS) in which electrodes were implanted via a surgical procedure near the dorsal column of the spinal cord and connecting wires passed subcutaneously to a receiver implanted commonly on the chest and back. When activated by the patient, electrical stimulation of the dorsal column resulted in altered feelings of tingling/paraesthesia in the pain site. , Complications, unfortunately, were common (McCaffery, 1979b).

The basic 'reasoning' of using cutaneous stimulation that closes the gate to the transmission of pain impulses is applied therapeutically by the non-invasive use of:

1. Heat
2. Cold
3. Massage
4. Transcutaneous electrical stimulation (TENS)

(See Non-Pharmacological Interventions, p. 144).

Endogenous Opiates

The potent effect of opium derivatives has been known for hundreds of years and they have been used clinically for their analgesic, calming, euphoriant and antidiarrhoeal properties; likewise, the consequence of opiate addiction in man has been profound and well documented.

The more recent identification of the morphine-like substances endorphins and enkephalins throughout the nervous system highlights the biochemical link of painful sensation and the sites of action of analgesics in neurotransmitters.

There exists in the literature a large and ever-increasing amount of information on the possible and probable functions of these endogenous opioid peptides, ranging widely from pain perception and analgesia, regulation of pancreatic secretion, respiration and eating, to learning behaviour, memory, and so on.

Similarly, there is mounting evidence to suggest that acupuncture and pain therapy involving electrical stimulation induce the release of endogenous opiates in both animals and humans (Pomeranz and Chui, 1976; Mayer and Price, 1977; Clement Jones *et al.*, 1980b).

Research findings suggest that endogenous opioid peptides may be activated by acupuncture, and that acupuncture analgesia is antagonized by naloxone, which reveals the involvement of opioid peptides in the process. Furthermore, there is evidence that the psychological and emotional state exerts influence on blood endorphin levels.

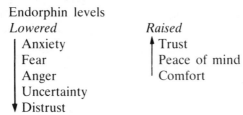

Endorphin levels

Lowered	*Raised*
Anxiety	Trust
Fear	Peace of mind
Anger	Comfort
Uncertainty	
Distrust	

This reduction in negative influences supports and assists the creation and maintenance of patients' own positive defence and coping mechanisms.

The early hope that endogenous peptides might be non-addictive and could replace opiates in pain relief has not been fulfilled. Animals treated with natural enkephalins demonstrate tolerance and dependence (Van Ree *et al.*, 1976). To date many enkephalin analogs have been synthesized and tested and, disappointingly, all have shown addictive properties.

Of the many opioid structures found in the body, substance P has the longest history; although known in 1934, it was not isolated until

1970 by Leeman. In 1977 in further studies Jessell and Iverson (1977) suggested a relationship between enkephalin and substance P, proposing this to be a physiologic/chemical basis for the 'pain gate' described by Melzack and Wall.

It is clear that endogenous opioids and their receptors have exciting and far-reaching implications for understanding the mechanisms and experience of pain. Through the provision of a biochemical link and structure for previous pain theories and individual variations in response to pain, mind and body can no longer be regarded as separate phenomena.

Psychophysiological Theories

The experience of pain has perceptive, reactive and evaluative components, described by Maclean (1975) in the 'triune' brain concept as an inner 'primitive' brain concerned with survival *sensory* functions, an intermediate level/limbic brain involved in *reactive* (emotional/ affective) functions and an outer advanced *evaluative* (cognitive) system concerned with conscious functions.

Sensory (perceptual) refers to the physical sensation of pain. This involves the sensory nerve pathways, spinothalamic tracts, thalamic nuclei and sensory cortex and does not require conscious awareness.

Reaction (affective/emotional) is the psychological and motivational response to pain and involves the limbic system in the basal region of the brain and cerebral cortex. The limbic system is involved in both autonomic and motor responses and is associated with sexual feelings, pleasure/sorrow, fear/anger.

Evaluative (cognitive) involves the higher centres of the cerebral cortex, i.e. is concerned with the interpretation of what pain means to the individual, and is dependent on culture, past pain experience, memory, personality and emotional state.

These three components contribute to the total dimension of pain, although at any given time the relative contribution of each may vary. Interventions that reduce the effect of them will help to relieve the severity of pain.

Summary of Relationships between Events in Pain Perception and Responses to the Experience of Pain

After a pain stimulus occurs it passes into the receptor state or nociception (Figure 1). This is where unpleasant (noxious) stimuli are

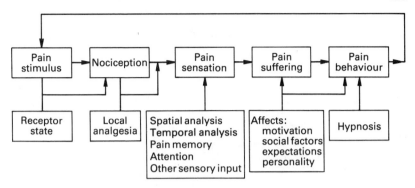

Figure 1. Summary of relationships in pain perception. The sequence of events between the initiation of pain and the resulting behaviour may be affected by the factors shown. Adapted from Loeser (1980), Melzack and Denis (1978) and Littlejohns and Vere (1981)

detected by receptors and converted into impulses carried by small fibre (A and C) afferent nerves to the cortex, where they are analysed as a pain sensation. At this stage the perception of pain will depend on the individual's interpretation of it. This will be expressed in terms of distress, pain suffering which will determine pain behaviour, i.e. individual response to pain.

1. The experience of pain is not a simple, straightforward response to an unpleasant sensation. It is a highly complex event involving many nerve pathways and mechanisms.
2. At its most basic level, it can be an immediate involuntary response disassociated from the complexities of perception and reaction.
3. Perception and response are dependent on other sensory inputs, motor activity, emotional state and past memory (Figure 2).

Perception and Reaction

Patients who have experienced a long illness, a series of operations or long-term distressing therapy, for example radiotherapy and cytotoxic drugs, may feel increasingly demoralized and experience mounting difficulties in contending with pain.

Some patients withdraw, others may call out, moan, weep, beg for help, become restless, pace up and down, toss and turn in bed or express thoughts of suicide. Whilst they may be recognized initially as individual reactions, cultural traditions, past environmental and parental

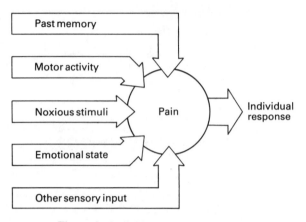

Figure 2. Individual response to pain

attitudes will mediate response to pain. In general, western culture does not encourage free expression of pain or emotion. Little children are discouraged from a very early age from crying and are told to be brave. Other cultures traditionally encourage a more spontaneous and open emotional response to life events. For example, the anthropologist Zborowski (1969) in his work on pain tolerance observed that people not only react to pain as individuals, but also their ethnic origins influence the way they react to and tolerate being in pain. He identified two behaviour states which he described as 'present orientated' and 'future orientated'. He found that 'old Americans' (descendants of Anglo-Saxon origin) had a matter-of-fact attitude to pain, with little outward expression, tending to withdraw when pain became intense. On the other hand, Jews and Italians were more expressive, seeking support and sympathy and crying out. Zborowski concluded that the Italians were 'present orientated', expressing appropriate concern about the presence of pain and seeking immediate relief. The Jews were 'future orientated'. While seeking immediate relief from their pain, they were also sceptical or suspicious of the future. They continued to complain despite diminution of pain severity and suffered 'future orientated anxiety'. The 'old Americans' shared the position of the Jews of 'future orientation', but were more optimistic. However, unlike both the Italians and the Jews, they tended to withdraw socially.

Understanding ethnic and cultural background is relevant in terms of assessment of pain and in understanding behavioural responses in both patients and staff. Differences of expression between cultural groups exist, and quite naturally each will consider their own behaviours and attitudes appropriate and correct.

Pain Threshold and Tolerance

There is considerable confusion in the use of the terms 'pain threshold' and 'pain tolerance', with assertions frequently being made that variations in pain expression between individuals are due to different pain thresholds. Melzack and Wall (1982) described four clearly identifiable specific levels of threshold.

- Sensation threshold (lower threshold), i.e. the lowest stimulus value at which a sensation such as tingling or warmth is first reported.
- Pain perception threshold, i.e. the lowest stimulus value at which the person reports that the stimulation is painful.
- Pain tolerance (upper threshold), i.e. the lowest stimulus level at which the subject withdraws or asks to have the stimulation stopped.
- Encouraged pain tolerance, i.e. the same as pain tolerance, but the person is encouraged to tolerate higher levels of stimulation.

Hardy, Wolff and Goodell (1952) and Sternbach and Tursky (1965) provided evidence that regardless of culture all people have a uniform sensation threshold. Similarly in 1977, Weisenberg in his review of the literature on cultural differences and pain perception suggested that these were due to differing cultural characteristics concerning the expression of pain rather than sensitivity differences.

Likewise differences of age, sex, personality, race and status between patients and staff are present; the potential role and influence of interactions between them have been described and their effect cannot be ignored (Davitz and Davitz, 1975; Hackett, 1971; Pilowsky and Bond, 1969).

Lewis (1978), discussing the relationship of culture to pain, emphasized two key areas. Our ability to sympathize with another person is dependent on our imaginative identification with him. Secondly we are less concerned by hurt to individuals we do not know, and as participants and observers an individual's pain experience affects and influences objectivity in pain assessment (Craig and Neidermayer, 1974; Craig and Prkachin, 1978; Krebs, 1975.)

Since so many naturally occurring behavioural variations exist in response to pain, the aim of care must be to:

1. Create a climate of acceptance, trust and understanding
2. Assume responsibility for pain relief and patients' comfort as a prime achievable goal
3. Not only have due regard and countenance for what is familiar, but equally respect and have compassion for that which is not ('care' has no brief for moral or cultural judgements).

The Significance of Pain

The presence of pain in seriously ill and dying patients will be a signal and constant reminder of the worsening of their condition, the passing of life and their approaching death. Any admission that pain exists does not convey the significance that the individual places upon it. Engel (1959) proposed that the significance placed upon pain could be outlined at three levels of symbolism of increasing complexity:

*   Pain may be a signal indicating danger to body structure
*   A situation may arise where two or more persons collectively complain thus forming a means of expressing a need for help.
*   As a complaint, pain may represent feelings of being unfairly treated or may be used as a way to manipulate others.

Pain may also become a vehicle that reflects feelings of guilt, which may become particularly highlighted in seriously ill and dying patients and as such come to be regarded as a punishment for real or imagined wrongdoing, evidenced by the Latin root *peona* and Greek *peine* meaning penalty and punishment.

This response may be seen in some religious attitudes to pain, suffering and death and may be felt as a means of close identification with God or as total rejection, with resultant feelings of distress, anger, bitterness and despair.

Pain Memory

The fear of uncontrolled pain at death may exceed the fears of death itself, and the relevance of past pain memory and experiences allied with misconceptions and unspoken anxieties cannot be ignored.

The brain has the capacity to reconstruct images of the past which have a powerful impact on the perception of the present. Goleman (1979) described this ability as analogous to the properties of a hologram, whereby a three-dimensional image of an object is produced by focusing light on a photographic plate previously exposed to a similar light. Such characteristics appear to be present in the brain, whereby a prior experience may be triggered and reproduced by a current experience with similar characteristics, thus accentuating and compounding the physical distress and emotional anguish experienced by patients suffering pain.

Communication and Pain

Patients have little power, and in a society that emphasizes youth and health the old, sick and dying may feel they have little place or importance, resulting in an inequality that directly affects communication. Tournier (1957) reflected 'when one dominates the other, there will no longer be a dialogue because one of the persons is eclipsed, his power of self-determination is paralysed'.

Most patients know when they are dying, whether or not they have been told, and many benefit from talking about it to those caring for them. Any 'conspiracy of silence' allows fears to grow and reticence in one area impedes communication and understanding about all else — particularly pain.

If pain remains uncontrolled, little else can be achieved.

A patient may expect that those that care for him will know all about his pain, assuming the pain to be 'typical' and therefore needing no further explanation. By the same token, the team may rely entirely on the patient 'telling' them about pain. Whilst direct conversation may be regarded as the most obvious form of contact, the greater part of the interactions between staff and patients are non-verbal.

Talking to patients can best be done by helping patients to relax, by sitting patiently and being ready to listen. Being seen to be 'busy' not only increases anxiety but results in poor, if not failure of, contact. Alternatively, persistent questioning and an 'inappropriate breeziness' in manner without giving time for answers stultifies response, manipulates the conversation and inhibits further discussion. This serves only the staff, who by their manner and actions control and keep all contact at its most superficial level and hasten away to the next problem and patient. Such behaviour thwarts and blocks the creation of an atmosphere in which trust and rapport can be established as the foundation of understanding patients' suffering and the total experience of pain.

Staff usually need to be alone with patients, seem unhurried, and use open-ended questions in order to receive and provide information in stages, as and when the patient is ready. Checks need to be made to ascertain what has been understood as fears and presuppositions may inhibit what is absorbed.

Communication involves not only speech but sensitivity, understanding and alertness to the signals of non-verbal cues in behaviour, posture and expression, namely:

- Changes in normal behaviour
- Marked withdrawal
- Restlessness/agitation
- Clenching of fists or teeth
- Facial grimacing
- Strained, drawn expression
- Sallow or greyish facial colour
- Sweating, cold and clammy skin
- Loss of appetite
- Rejection of company
- Excessive fatigue and lassitude
- Mood change

Unrelieved Pain

A century ago 5 per cent of deaths occurred in hospital. The proportion is now estimated to be 60 per cent overall, 70 per cent in urban areas, with 65.4 per cent of all cancer deaths occurring in hospital (Lunt, 1980).

General improvement in health and social care provision has meant that people are living longer, with one-third potentially outliving relatives to care for them. Within this group the incidence of neoplastic disease is steadily rising.

Despite the achievement of 'hospice type' care over the past decade, notably in the relief of pain and control of distressing symptoms, there is little evidence of systematic teaching of these in medical and nursing schools or in the curriculum of other health care professionals. Bonica (1980) in his review of the reasons for 'non-relief' suggested that the most important cause was the improper application of current knowledge and lack of observation and assessment skills. This statement is reflected and underwritten by accumulative and disturbing results of a series of studies revealing evidence of:

- Unrelieved pain
- Poor symptom control
- Social isolation
- Mental and physical distress
- Rising bed occupancy

Lunt (1980) observed that 70 per cent of people die in hospital, and whilst dying patients may spend two-thirds of the last months of life at home, many are admitted to hospital to die because of lack of facilities and support at home (Bowling, 1982).

Admission to hospital, however, has been no guarantee of effective symptom control and psychological support (Cartwright, Hockey and Anderson, 1973). Studies of seriously ill and dying patients have revealed serious shortcomings in patient care and family support (Bowling and Cartwright, 1982).

Hockley (1983) in a study of 26 dying patients found evidence of unrelieved symptoms; on occasions medical and nursing staff were unaware of patients suffering sleepless nights, mouth infection, persistent and at times distressing pain. Hunt et al. (1978) in a study of protracted pain revealed staff underestimation of pain and site involvement, poor communication and the presence of unrelieved pain.

In earlier work Hinton (1963) described dying patients' feelings of isolation, anxiety and depression, indicating a significant lack of psychological and emotional support and of understanding by staff of the nature and depth of patients' needs.

Twycross and Fairfield (1982) found that 73 out of 100 patients admitted to a hospice had pain for more than eight weeks and 57 for more than sixteen weeks, and of the 73 patients, over three-quarters described their pain as severe, very severe or excruciating.

Parkes (1978) in his study of community patients interviewed the surviving spouses of cancer patients; their memory one year after the patient's death revealed a high incidence of 'severe and mostly continuous pain' during both the preterminal and terminal phase and that the incidence of unrelieved pain rose sharply from 6 per cent preterminally to 28 per cent in the terminal phase.

Marks and Sachar (1973) and Hunt et al. (1978) produced supporting evidence that pain is often inadequately relieved. More recently, Twycross estimated that of the two-thirds of cancer patients who experience severe pain from their illness, 25 per cent of all cancer patients, that is 30 000, die without relief from severe pain in the United Kingdom each year.

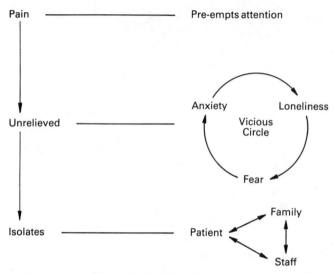

Figure 3. Unrelieved pain

The implications of this are not only immediately apparent for patients in terms of misery and suffering but also for their families who witness and share their experiences and the staff who are responsible for their care — few can remain unaffected (Figure 3).

The reasons for unrelieved pain are both complex and varied, and in a series of studies conducted at The London Hospital eight main problem areas emerged (Raiman, 1986). (See Table 1.)

Response

1. To respond effectively to pain, goals need to be set and care planned individually.
2. All interrelating factors must be taken into account that actively reflect patients' needs and which provide information on the pain.
3. '*Listening*' to patients provides the vital link between the components that influence response:
   (i) Physical and pathological causes of pain (Table 2)
   (ii) Factors influencing response to pai (Table 3)
   (iii) Factors which modify the pain threshold (Table 4)
   (iv) Common symptoms which influence the response to pain (Table 5)
   (v) Characteristics of and differences between acute and chronic pain (Table 6)

Table 1. Reasons for unrelieved pain

Low expectation of relief
    Lack of understanding   Drug tolerance
    lack of knowledge   Drug dependence
    Fear   Drug adverse effect
    Stoicism, 'brave face'
    Fatalism, pain is 'inevitable/untreatable'

Inadquate treatment skills, inadequate drug utilization
    Choice, dose, frequency of drug
    Adverse effects/lack of adjuvant prescribing
    As-required prescribing
    Non-use co-analgesics (e.g. NSAID)
    Mixed prescribing,   Agonist
       lowering total analgesic   Partial agonists
       effect   Antagonist

Low treatment aims
    Pain does not exist
    Pain does not matter
    Pain is acceptable

Non-drug scotoma
    Position, massage, physical aids
    Time, support, distraction
    Palliative radiotherapy

Inadequate account of pain
    Poor comprehension of mechanism(s) of pain(s)
    Underestimation of sites, severity
    Nature/meaning of pain
    Lack of patient involvement

Inadequate monitoring
    Inflexibility
    No systematic observation
    Lack of patient involvement

Communication
    Absent
    Distant
    Clumsy
    Poor doctor–nurse cooperation

Administrative delays
    Indecision   Delays in
    Dithering   pain control

Table 2. Physical and pathological causes of pain

Genetic
Personality
Ethnic
Cultural
Environmental
Experience
Socioeconomic

Table 3. Factors influencing response to pain

Threshold lowered	Threshold raised
Insomnia	Sleep
Fatigue	Rest
Anxiety	Sympathy
Fear	Understanding
Anger	Diversion
Sadness	Elevation of mood
Depression	Analgesics
Mental isolation	Antidepressants
Introversion	Axiolytics
Past experience	

Table 4. Factors which modify the pain threshold

Anorexia
General malaise and lassitude
Constipation
Diarrhoea
Nausea and vomiting
Cough
Dyspnoea
Inflammation
Oedema
Immobility
Anxiety and fear
Depression
Dryness of the mouth and fungal
  infections

Table 5. Common symptoms of disease which influence the response to pain

Infiltration of nerve, blood vessels and periosteum by tumour cells
Compression of nerves by tumour mass
Infection
Inflammation and necrosis
Ischaemia
Distension of pelvic and abdominal viscera, lymphoedema
Malignant ascites and effusion, elevated intracranial pressure
Venous thrombosis and pulmonary embolism
Ulceration

Table 6. Differences between acute and chronic pain. Data after Twycross (1976)

	Acute pain	Chronic pain
Conduction pathways	Rapid	Slow
Tissue injury	Clearly causal	Minor or absent
Automatic response	Present	Absent
Biological value	High	Low
Mood	Anxiety	Depression, anxiety
Social effects	Slight	Marked
Effective treatment	Analgesics	Variable, sometimes none

4. Acute pain has a meaning. Its presence can be seen as a signal or warning that prompts action and remedial relief. It is usually of limited duration and the social and psychological effects are slighter.
5. Conversely, chronic, unrelieved, continuous pain is intensified by its lack of meaning. It disrupts every living day and if unrelieved destroys patients' confidence and trust.

Summary

- Pain is detrimental
- Pain has physical, psychological, spiritual, social and environmental components
- Acute and chronic pain require different treatment approaches

- Unrelieved pain isolates, and creates a vicious circle, with anxiety, depression and fear. This may lead staff to avoid contact with the patient, at a time when the need for reassurance, comfort and positive action is increasing
- The experience of pain is individual, with no known 'correct levels' of intensity, suffering or response to treatment. The 'between patient' response can also be reflected as a 'within patient reaction', i.e. an individual patient's ability to respond and contend with pain will alter and change from time to time. The intensity levels of pain may also vary considerably during the day and night.

Intervention

A *treatment plan* for pain comprises some or all of the following:

(i) Pharmacological interventions
(ii) Non-pharmacological interventions.

Pharmacological Interventions

Analgesia

The word analgesia is derived from the Greek words *An — without* and *Algos — pain.*

Action of Analgesics

Analgesics act upon the nervous system by affecting perceptual mechanisms. In addition, narcotic drugs alter the emotional response to pain (cortical action). At the peripheral level, the production of pain-producing substances in the tissues such as kinins and prostaglandins is interfered with by the use of drugs such as salicylates, aspirin being the most common.

1. *Assessment*
    Analgesic relief should be assessed in relation to comfort achieved throughout the 24-hour period:
    (i)   At night
    (ii) During the day
    (iii) On movement
    (iv) At rest

2. Reassessment
    This is particularly needed for patients with chronic multifocal
    pain. 'Old pains may get worse, and new ones emerge.' Review is
    essential.
3. Evaluation
    Regular detailed evaluation on the efficiency of analgesics following
    administration should take place, as follows:
    (i)   How long does it take for the drugs to work?
    (ii) How much relief is achieved?
    (iii) How long does the relief last?
    (iv) Be alert for side-effects
    (v)   Observe and report accurately
4. Patient participation
    This should be:
         Sought
         Encouraged
         Respected
         Believed

Analgesia: Basic Principles

It is essential to have a thorough understanding of the various types
of analgesics and the basic principles underlying and governing their
use, e.g.

- Duration of action
- Potency
- Toxicity and side-effects
- Agonists and antagonists
- Efficacy
- Cumulation
- Tolerance
- Dependence

Also essential is appreciation that chronic pain needs regular
analgesia, e.g. each dose is given before the pain returns; 'as-required'
prescribing is not compatible with protracted pain, except to make
available additional adjuvant analgesics to boost and enhance the
regular doses.

1. *Individual variation*
    There is a wide range of individual variation at any age, but
    particularly sensitive are the very young or older patients.

2. *Duration of action*

   Drugs vary in length of time within which they act, i.e. remain effective. For example, morphine and diamorphine are short-acting drugs; the half-life of their analgesic effect is between two and four hours. This follows closely the plasma drug concentration. The aim is to maintain the plasma level of the analgesic in the therapeutic 'usual effect' band but below that of toxicity.

3. *Efficacy*

   This is the maximum effect a given dose will produce. In severe pain only opiates and opioids have sufficient efficacy.

4. *Potency*

   This is a comparison of doses (milligramme to milligramme) between two similarly acting drugs.

5. *Toxicity*

   This is a level at which drugs cause unwanted effects; for example, aspirin can cause tinnitus and gastric bleeding, opiates/opioids constipation, nausea and vomiting.

6. *Cumulation*

   This is the gradual build-up and storage of a drug in the tissues. For example, the metabolism of methadone is complex and it has a far longer half-life than that of morphine or diamorphine and remains in the body for a greater period of time.

7. *Tolerance*

   This occurs only when the body becomes used to a drug and progressively larger doses are needed to maintain pain relief. Fortunately, this does not inevitably produce toxicity, for if tolerance occurs the level at which side-effects become a problem rises in proportion.

8. *Dependence*

   Physical dependence will develop with patients receiving opiates, i.e. drugs that exhibit tolerance also produce dependence. This is not the same as addiction, which has a very strong link with drug abuse and a psychological component. Even after long-term use, opiates can be tapered off and withdrawn if this is clinically appropriate.

9. *Agonists, partial agonists, antagonists*

   Opiate and opioid drugs* differ in their affinity to bind with the opiate receptors in the brain, a series of highly complex mechanisms.

---

* *Opiate* is a naturally occurring alkaloid of the poppy; *opioid* is a synthetic morphine-like substance.

Pure agonists: morphine and diamorphine
Partial agonists: pentazocine and codeine
Antagonists: naloxone and naltroxone

In practical terms, using a mixture of pure agonists with partial agonists will decrease analgesic effect, whilst antagonists will reverse the action of pure agonists (which, whilst preventing pain relief, can be used to reverse the side-effects of respiratory depression).

Summary

See Figures 4–9. For text of summary, see pp. 140 and 141.

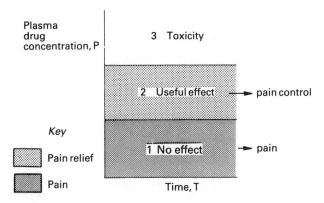

Figure 4. Plasma concentration zone in relation to drug effects. (Key to Figures 5–8 also)

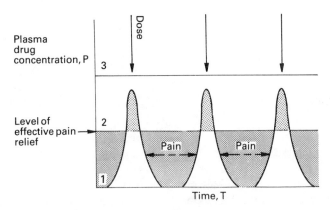

Figure 5. Short-acting drugs

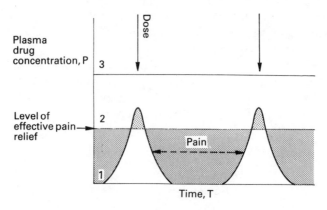

Figure 6. Overspaced doses or 'as-required' analgesia

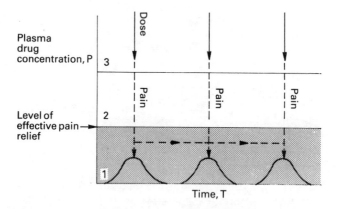

Figure 7. Doses too small to achieve pain relief. NB: Giving analgesia does not automatically produce pain relief

1. *Regular analgesia* given in such doses and at such times that pain does not recur, with supplements available for particular occasions such as nursing or medical procedures.
2. *Co-analgesia*, using drugs to relieve pain by other than a direct analgesic mechanism, e.g.:
   (a) a non-steroidal anti-inflammatory drug to inhibit the local production of prostaglandins, which sensitize free nerve endings and induce bone destruction.

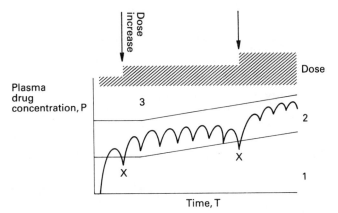

Figure 8. The effects of tolerance. Dosage is increased at X to maintain pain control as tolerance occurs

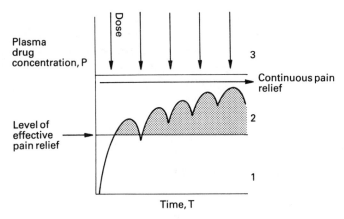

Figure 9. Doses spaced at satisfactory intervals to maintain analgesia. In chronic pain (such as in cancer) analgesia must be given regularly throughout the 24-hr period to achieve continuous pain relief

(b) a corticosteroid to reduce capillary permeability and peritumor oedema, and so diminish the headache of raised intracranial pressure and the pain of nerve compression or extensive soft tissue infiltration.

(c) an antibiotic to treat painful infections, e.g. infected ulcers.

3. *Adjuvant drug therapy* to offset the adverse effects of analgesics which might otherwise limit the acceptable dose.

Which Analgesic?

It may help to visualize analgesics in a 'league table' in three categories corresponding to mild, moderate and severe pain:

1. *Mild analgesics*, e.g. aspirin, paracetamol.
2. *Intermediate analgesics* (partial agonists). Weaker group — codeine, dihydrocodeine, or nefopam and meptazinol (not strictly opioids).
3. *Strong analgesics* (full agonists). Morphine, diamorphine, sometimes phenazocine, methadone, levorphanol (pethidine is too short-acting to be of use for chronic pain). NB. In addition, full agonists are usually made less effective by the addition of a partial agonist.

Dose and Timing

- Regular doses are given throughout the 24-hour period to prevent persistent pain returning and so diminish the fear of pain.
- An analgesic given only 'as required' to patients with persistent pain means that before each dose the patient will have to suffer pain and the allied anxiety that could have been avoided.
- 'As-required' analgesic can be a useful *addition* to a *regular* regimen, and occasionally may be all the analgesia needed by a patient who has pain only intermittently.

Route

- Most patients require only oral medication. However, oral medication may become inappropriate in the presence of dysphagia or nausea/intractable vomiting despite an antiemetic.
- Suppositories can be useful and avoid the need for injection (morphine in various strengths, and oxycodone are the strong analgesics available in this form).
- Injections of opiates may be needed, particularly in the initial control of overwhelming pain or in the last few days or hours of life (diamorphine as ampoules is particularly suitable for use by injection, being the only opiate soluble enough to allow low volume of injections).

Syringe Driver Pump

When patients cannot swallow or when bowel function is impaired the need for repeated injections can be obviated by the use of a compact portable syringe driver. The diamorphine is given continuously via a subcutaneous butterfly needle. (The use of diamorphine alone may be preferred or a mixture of diamorphine and antiemetic agents.) Skin reactions are more prone to occur with added phenothiazines, e.g. prochlorperazine. Each day's dosage is newly made up to avoid infection. The needle site need not be changed unless there is tissue reaction or swelling.

Principal Unwanted Effects

Constipation always occurs in patients taking morphine-like drugs. Nausea also occurs in many patients. Tolerance to nausea and vomiting usually develops and antiemetic therapy can often be discontinued after a week or so. These unwanted actions should be anticipated and offset from the start by using appropriate therapy.

Myths

For many years there have been unfounded fears concerning the use of morphine, now replaced by the facts that:

(i) Adequate analgesia with opioids does not significantly shorten the lifespan of patients with advanced cancer.
(ii) Physical dependence prevents sudden dose reduction, but psychological dependence ('addiction') is not a problem; if other measures relieve pain, the opiate dose can be reduced or even stopped.
(iii) Tolerance with a rising dose to achieve the same effect is not a problem; on average, the dose needed slowly reaches a plateau within about twelve weeks or earlier.
(iv) Sedation is common only in the first two to three days of a regular opiate; thereafter adequate analgesia is compatible with full mobility and a varied life.
(v) Pain stimulates the respiratory centre so opiates do not cause dangerous respiratory depression (even in respiratory disease, provided the dose is carefully titrated against the pain).

General Comment

Effective analgesia can almost always be attained, but attention should always be directed to the 'whole' person and to the whole clinical environment.

Side-effects can be avoided.

Drug therapy should be used as part of a pattern of total care.

If pain remits, opiates can be withdrawn readily provided this is done by gradual dose reduction.

Non-Pharmacological Interventions

Primary Intervention

Primary interventions are aimed at eliminating or reducing the cause of pain and include surgery, nerve blocks, radiotherapy and chemotherapy.

Unrelieved 'intractable' pain such as the pain of nerve compression and tumour infiltration may be helped by such techniques as:

1. Rhizotomy (nerve bocks) in which the pain is 'blocked' before the sensory route enters the spinal cord.
2. Cordotomy in which sensory pathways in the spinal cord are cut (relieving pain below the operative site).
3. Pituitary ablation.

Secondary Intervention

Secondary interventions are aimed at eliminating or reducing the pain intensity or, by increasing the pain tolerance of patients (McCaffery, 1979b), enhancing their ability to cope with it.

Physical comfort

Thoughtful planned anticipatory care using physical intervention and techniques can improve the quality of patients' day-to-day living, e.g.:

- Heat pads
- Cold packs
- Warm baths
- Additional support, e.g. immobilization by collar, splints or traction
- Special beds to assist movement and minimize handling together with additional aids:
     Sheepskin pads
     Additional pillows
     Ripple mattress

Cradle
Back rest
- Mouth care (crushed ice to suck, warm gargles, lipsalve)
- Relief of abdominal and bladder distension
- Careful positioning before turning/moving, with particular support to painful areas (muscles become cramped if in one position too long and pressure becomes pain over a long period)

Transcutaneous nerve stimulation

Historical accounts exist on the use of externally applied electrical stimulation for over a hundred years (South American Indians are known to have used electric eels to relieve pain).

Head and Rivers (1920) were among the first authors to refer to 'input' control, and although ablative measures can and are used they are invasive, may not be wholly successful and all carry a certain degree of morbidity.

Following the publication of the 'gate control' theory, the use of lower intensity stimulation selectively to activate the large diameter nerve fibres and 'close the gate' at the spinal or higher levels was recognized to have therapeutic potential in the relief of pain (Wall and Sweet, 1967).

The improvement of electrode materials and the miniaturization of the stimulation equipment has made TNS a practical adjuvant proposition in the management of chronic pain (Ostrowski, 1977).

Massage

Touch, pressure, stroking, massage, cryokinetics (ice massage), mentholated rubs, have been found to be helpful and comforting by different groups of patients with varying diagnoses from musculoskeletal conditions to cancer (Grant, 1964; Fraser, 1978; De Crosta, 1984).

Their mode of action is unclear, but various theories have been proposed:

1. Stimulation of the 'C' fibres helps to compete with the 'A delta' fibres carrying messages of sharp pain.
2. Stimulation activates the release of enkephalin in the CNS. Similarly, the technique of *acupuncture* is thought to work through the release of endorphins.

3. Stimulation effectively closes the 'gate' (Melzack and Wall, 1965) to the transmission of pain sensation.
4. Stimulation may increase/decrease blood supply, which will promote muscle relaxation and assist control of oedema.

'Touch' almost above all else, can demonstrate care, empathy and concern.

Entonox

In the 1960s a mixture of 50 per cent nitrous oxide with 50 per cent oxygen using a demand valve apparatus (Entonox) was introduced for the use of patients in labour. Its value in the relief of acute pain has now been acknowledged and it is becoming widely used to relieve the 'inflicted' pain of investigations and nursing/medical procedures (Diggory and Tiffany, 1979).

Relaxation strategies

Relaxation helps reduce muscle tension and anxiety. The relaxation response in man consists of changes opposite to those of the 'fight or flight response' (Wallace and Benson, 1972; Benson, 1975). This appears to be an integrated hypothalamic response resulting in decreased sympathetic nervous system activity with some increased parasympathetic response.

Physiological changes occurring during the practice of various techniques which elicit the relaxation response are:

Decreased	Increased
Oxygen consumption	Skin resistance
Respiratory rate	EEG alpha wave activity
Heart rate	
Muscle tension	

Meditation techniques have existed for centuries in practically all cultures, usually within a religious context; they allow an individual to experience the relaxation response within an altered state of consciousness.

Therapeutic intervention

Distraction helps break the 'tension, anxiety' cycle and relieve the sense of isolation experienced by patients with unrelieved pain by:

- Activating personal coping mechanisms
- 'Placing' pain out at the edge of awareness.

Various methods are used to:

- Promote progressive muscle relaxation (PMR)
- Enhance feelings of control.

Thus, whilst its presence may remain, attention is drawn towards focusing on other sensations and thoughts and the experience of pain is modulated.

Methods
Imagery,
Biofeedback
Hypnosis
Autogenic training
Yoga
Zen
Massage
Breathing techniques
Auditory stimulation:
   music
   radio/television

(Donovan, 1980; Connally, 1985)

Pain is at its most destructive when it dominates and nullifies all else. We need to help patients shift their focus of attention and concentration away from pain in order that its existence becomes *less important* in dealing with it effectively than developing strategies and enhancing positive attitudes towards coping with it and *diminishing its effect*.

Evaluation

'The simplest and most reliable index of pain is the patient's verbal report' (Lasagna, 1960).

It is a matter of considerable professional concern that for so many years observation and assessment of pain has remained a largely neglected area. As with all other treatment and care, pain requires a problem-solving analytical approach which should aim to:

1. Provide an accurate *pain profile* and history.
2. Establish *observation and assessment* interventions.

Pain Profile

A series of straightforward questions will immediately help to establish essential facts about the pain.

1. ، Time (*past*)
    (i)   When did the pain begin (hours, days, weeks, months, years)?
    (ii) Under what circumstances did it occur?
    Time (*present*)
    (iii) When do you get the pain?

        Daily
            (a) during the day:
            (b) at night, how often does this occur?
            (c) on movement, e.g. standing, walking, bending, etc.?
            (d) at rest?

        Weekly or occasionally each month?

    Diurnal variation
    (iv) Have you noticed any particular 'pattern' to your pain, e.g. is it worse at any particular time during the 24 hours?
2. Location (*site(s)*)
    (i)   Where is the pain?
    (ii) Does it remain in one place, or does it change, and if so where and when?
3. *Nature*
    What does your pain feel like? (e.g. dull, burning, shooting)?
4. *Relief*
    Is there anything that helps your pain?
5. *Coping*
    Is there anything that you do that you find helps with the pain?
6. *Effect*
    (i) *Activities*
    Does the pain interfere with your day-to-day activities
        (a) at home?

    (b)   at work?
    (c)   socially?
(ii)   *Emotion*
    (a)   Does your pain change if you are feeling low, worried or
          tense?
    (b)   Does your pain change if you are occupied?
    (c)   Does your pain change if you are relaxed/enjoying
          yourself?
(iii) *Treatment*
       Have you had any treatment that has had an effect upon your
       pain?
    (a)   Medication:
          painkillers?
          other medication?
    (b)   Surgical treatment
    (c)   Nerve blocks
    (d)   Physiotherapy (e.g. heat, massage, exercises)
    (e)   Any other forms of activity/intervention (e.g. acupuncture,
          relaxation, etc., etc.)

Measurement of pain

A slow but steady stream of information has accumulated from
researchers and clinicians over the past 40 years in the development
and use of 'tools' to measure and assess pain in both laboratory and
clinical settings.

Besides questionnaires using both scaled and open-ended questions,
various tools and scales have been developed and tested (Huskisson,
1974; Scott and Huskisson, 1976; Woodford and Merksey, 1972;
Reading, 1980; Downie *et al.*, 1978; Aitken, 1969; McGuire, 1984;
Lasagna, 1960).

Verbal descriptor scales (verbal rating scales)

These scales consist of three to five numerically ranked choice of word
descriptors, e.g. none, slight, mild, moderate, severe.

The number corresponding to the word chosen is used to determine
the severity of the pain. The first known use was by Keele (1948), who
developed and used a pain chart for the assessment of surgical pain,
angina and gastrointestinal ulcers.

Visual analogues scales

These scales consist of a 10 cm line which represents a 'continuum of intensity' and has verbal anchors at either end (Maxwell, 1978), e.g.

No pain ◄──────────────────────► Pain as bad as it could be

                                10 cm

Patients are asked to 'mark' their pain along this line at a point between the two extremes which represents the level of their pain and the result is measured in millimetres.

Other measurement techniques

Other methods have been developed that attempt to match the intensity of patients' perceived pain to some other quantifiable entity such as behavioural or physiological response to pain.

   Instruments have been developed that measure more than these two dimensions in an effort to produce a more complete measurement of the experience of pain. (Johnson, 1972, 1973; Johnson and Rice, 1974; Melzack and Torgerson 1971; Daut, Cleeland and Flanery, 1983). Of these the McGill Pain Questionnaire (Melzack, 1975) and the Wisconsin Brief Pain Questionnaire (Daut, Cleeland and Flanery, 1983) are the most widely used.

   In 1981 Bourbonnais developed and tested a 'pain ruler' combining rating scales and word descriptors for use by nurses with patients suffering acute and chronic pain.

Observation and Assessment

Over a period of years the author has worked with seriously ill and dying patients with pain, their families and staff.

   Though entering sensitive and emotive areas, it has been possible to study in a scientific and valid way their needs, outline some of the reasons for non-relief (see Table 1), and in response develop methods to improve pain control and aid communication in hospital and at home (Raiman, 1986b, c). (See Figure 10 (pp. 153–5), The London Hospital Pain Chart, and Figure 11 (pp. 156–7), The London Hospital Home Diary.)

   Table 7 indicates the principles of assessment and observation.

Table 7. Principles of assessment and observation

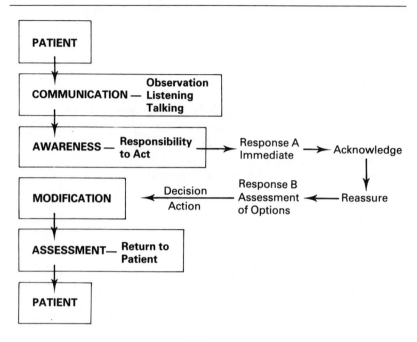

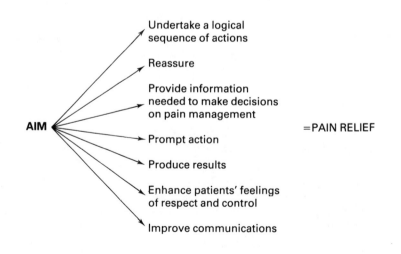

Care has been taken to provide a balance between *expression* using body outlines, *systematic review* and *individual measures* to:

1. Improve communications between patient, nurse and doctor by systematizing the recording of pain regularly.
2. Focus attention on the mechanisms of different pains and provide information on what relieves them, by recording each site separately.
3. To have readily available in one place information that is useful in making decisions about the management of pain.
4. Bring together skills, knowledge and coping mechanisms to aid and encourage individual assessment.
5. Achieve a system to be used *with* patients and *not* on or to them.

Discussion

Patients

People who experience unrelieved pain over a period of time enter an alien, frightening world. Where the normal framework of time limit, sense of control and remedial action is overturned and replaced by feelings of despair, helplessness and vulnerability, and in an attempt to give 'meaning' to their experience, personal feelings of guilt and collective cultural reactions become aroused.

Unable to sleep, patients may withdraw, become anxious, and feel increasingly isolated from all around them, losing trust in both family and staff. Staff too react, ward rounds hurry by, side wards are used, and in this atmosphere patient and family 'leavetaking' is marred and the pattern of normal grieving potentially arrested and damaged.

Clinical Review

Assessment of pain is no different in principle or practice to the assessment of all other patient care problems — and its successful implementation is the key to all other care.

Without a clear plan that includes an individual pain history/profile and a firm commitment to participative observation and assessment, it becomes increasingly difficult for staff to return time and again to a patient with mounting needs if there exists a shared sense of 'helplessness', loss of morale and lack of information from which to evaluate and modify treatment and care.

A clear plan needs to be formulated detailing:

- Overall aims and objectives of care
- Assessment of the pain profile (site, severity, nature, effect)
- Individual coping mechanisms
- Interventions/pain relief measures
    Pharmacological
    Non-pharmacological
- Evaluation of intervention effectiveness (systematic observation and assessment of the pain with the patient)

THE LONDON HOSPITAL PAIN OBSERVATION CHART

Pain is a wholly subjective symptom. In consequence, there is no easy way of understanding what a patient is suffering, nor of conveying information about it from one person to another, though doctors and nurses need to do so. For instance, a doctor who needs to check the effectiveness of an analgesic prescription may find it difficult to say what information should be decisive. Thus, problems of communication can result in poor control of pain.

The pain observation chart is intended to improve communication between patient, nurse and doctor by making the recording of pain more systematic; the idea owes a lot to charts for neurological observations. Secondly, it is intended to make readily available in one place the information that is useful when taking decisions about the management of pain; for this reason some information already available on the drug chart, and some in the nursing record is inevitably duplicated in it. Thirdly, it is intended to focus attention on the mechanisms of different pains, and to provide evidence on what relieves them, by recording each site of pain separately.

You are likely to find this chart most useful when you know that a patient's pain is a problem, or you think it may be. It is a means of communication, to be used with the patient, not on the patient. Nurses should have it available at the handover report between shifts, and doctors will need it for ward rounds. The brief comments allowed may prove unexpectedly significant, and need amplification, so it is important that each entry is initialled. Occasionally, it may be a good idea to have two separate, independent charts, one kept by the patient, the other by the staff.

Figure 10. The London Hospital Pain Observation Chart. (Figure continues on pp. 154 and 155)

THIS CHART records where a patient's pain is and how bad it is, by the nurse asking the patient at regular intervals. If analgesics are being given regularly, make an observation <u>with</u> each dose and another <u>half-way between</u> each dose. If analgesics are given only 'as required', observe two-hourly. When the observations are stable and the patient is comfortable, any regular time interval between observations may be chosen.

DATE ....

SHEET
NUMBER ....

TO USE THIS CHART ask the patient to mark all his or her pains on the body diagram below. Label each site of pain with a letter (ie. A, B, C etc).

Then at each observation time ask the patient to assess:

1   The **pain in each separate site** since the last observation.
    Use the scale above the body diagram, and enter the number or letter in the appropriate column.

2   The **pain overall** since the last observation. Use the same scale and enter in column marked OVERALL.

Next, record what has been done to relieve pain:

3   Note any **analgesic** given since the last observation – stating name, dose, route, and time given.

4   Tick any other **nursing care or action** taken to ease pain.

Finally, note any **comment** on pain from patient or nurse (use the back of the chart as well, if necessary) and initial the record.

Excruciating	5
Very severe	4
Severe	3
Moderate	2
Just noticeable	1
No pain at all	0
Patient sleeping	S

TIME	PAIN RATING

BY SITES OVER-
A B C D E F G H ALL

Left   Right   Right   Left

Figure 10 cont'd

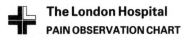
The London Hospital
PAIN OBSERVATION CHART

PATIENT
IDENTIFICATION
LABEL

ANALGESIC GIVEN (Name, dose, route, time)	Lifting	Turning	Massage	Distracting activities *	Position change *	Additional aids *	Other *	COMMENTS FROM PATIENTS AND/OR STAFF	Initials

MEASURES TO RELIEVE PAIN   Specify where starred

Figure 10 cont'd

HOME DIARY

L H M C

NAME ....

DATE STARTED ....

Please fill in body outline to show where your pains are

Right   Left   Left   Right

Right   Left

This is a diary about your pain.
Please fill it in daily to show:
how well you have slept
the pain killers you take
how bad your pain is
any different pain, symptom or
unusual activity/exercise

	ANY OTHER COMMENTS	NOTES of any different pain, symptom or problem, and any unusual activity or exercise during each day
Day 1		
Day 2		
Day 3		
Day 4		
Day 5		
Day 6		
Day 7		

HOW TO FILL IN THE HOME DIARY

1 Sleep: In this column, fill in hours slept, then ring word which best describes how much your pain disturbed your rest.

2 Pain: In the column for each day, write the number of doses of painkiller (tablets, spoonfuls) taken. Then choose the best word to describe your pain for that part of the day. Put in the chart the pain number next to the word you chose.

3 On the back of the diary, make a note of any different pains, symptoms, or problems and note any unusual activities of exercise that day.

4 Add any other comments of your own.

		Excruciating	5
		Very severe	4
		Severe	3
		Moderate	2
		Just noticeable	1
		No pain at all	0

	SLEEP	MORNING (to 12 noon)	AFTERNOON (noon to 4 pm)	EARLY EVENING (4 to 8 pm)	LATE EVENING (from 8 pm)
Day 1	Hours of sleep / Pain disturbed sleep never/a bit/often/a lot	No. of pain killers / Pain number	No. of pain killers / Pain number	No. of pain killers / Pain number	No. of pain killers / Pain number
Day 2	Hours of sleep / Pain disturbed sleep never/a bit/often/a lot	No. of pain killers / Pain number	No. of pain killers / Pain number	No. of pain killers / Pain number	No. of pain killers / Pain number
Day 3	Hours of sleep / Pain disturbed sleep never/a bit/often/a lot	No. of pain killers / Pain number	No. of pain killers / Pain number	No. of pain killers / Pain number	No. of pain killers / Pain number
Day 4	Hours of sleep / Pain disturbed sleep never/a bit/often/a lot	No. of pain killers / Pain number	No. of pain killers / Pain number	No. of pain killers / Pain number	No. of pain killers / Pain number
Day 5	Hours of sleep / Pain disturbed sleep never/a bit/often/a lot	No. of pain killers / Pain number	No. of pain killers / Pain number	No. of pain killers / Pain number	No. of pain killers / Pain number
Day 6	Hours of sleep / Pain disturbed sleep never/a bit/often/a lot	No. of pain killers / Pain number	No. of pain killers / Pain number	No. of pain killers / Pain number	No. of pain killers / Pain number
Day 7	Hours of sleep / Pain disturbed sleep never/a bit/often/a lot	No. of pain killers / Pain number	No. of pain killers / Pain number	No. of pain killers / Pain number	No. of pain killers / Pain number

Figure 11. The London Hospital Home Diary

Future Priorities

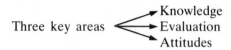

Three key areas → Knowledge / Evaluation / Attitudes

There is a clear personal and professional requirement on clinicians, managers, educators and researchers to accept responsibility for the relief of pain.

- A detailed knowledge base exists on the place and use of:

— Analgesics and co-analgesia
— Hormone therapy
— Neurosurgery
— Nerve-block techniques
— Palliative radiotherapy

- There is a greater understanding and growing awareness of the use of non-pharmacological measures and strategies to relieve pain
- Observation and assessment tools and methods have been developed and evaluated
- Specialist Macmillan nurses exist as clinical and education resources

1. Knowledge

The first priority is to absorb and fully integrate into everyday practice and care the knowledge and resources that exist.

2. Evaluation

The second is to undertake continuing forms of assessment and evaluation on the needs of seriously ill and dying patients and their families, together with studies to establish and inform in what circumstances, and for whom, one form of treatment/approach/care undertaken to relieve pain is judged to be more appropriate or preferable to others.

It is no longer enough simply to 'feel and say that is so'.

3. Attitudes

The third is a more elusive challenge.

Society's interest and concern in health and health care provision is greater than at any time previously.

This awareness leads to heightened expectations and a natural questioning on the appropriateness of the traditional staff — patient relationship, with its potential imbalance of professional dominance over compliant, passive patients and clients.

It remains to be seen how and to what extent professionals are able to respond to and accept patient participation and involvement in the choice of:

(1) The treatment modality
(2) The setting of care
(3) The establishment of outcome goals
(4) The observation and assessment of pain

Not all patients will wish or be capable of participating in assessing their pain and planning for its relief. Indeed some may see such actions and decisions resting entirely with the staff who care for them. Nor will all staff have the motivation, sensitivity and communication skills to foster and encourage patient participation.

As early as 1956 Szasz and Hollender proposed three models of staff–patient relationships: activity–passivity, guidance–cooperation, and mutual participation. The first model applies with a comatose patient; such a patient is by definition passive, i.e. completely helpless, and the staff assume an authoritative role. The second model applies to acute patients who can actively cooperate with the regimen outlined. In the third model, staff 'help the patient to help himself' and the patient is regarded as an equal in the delivery of care. This model has particular relevance for patients with long-term or advanced disease where from the patient's perspective, pain and illness rob them of valued aspects of life such as self-determination and individual identity.

As Brody (1980) suggests, this approach is not intended to compel patients to participate in every trivial decision, nor is it a method by which staff abdicate responsiblity by forcing patients into an inappropriate and untenable position of 'self care'. 'Mutual participation' offers an opportunity for a relationship to develop whereby patients feelings of self-esteem and control are enhanced and their values and wishes are preserved. This is the optimum base upon which decisions are made.

> 'Not only degrees of pain but its existence must be taken upon the testimony of the patient'.
>
> Peter Mere Latham (1789–1875)

Extracts from this chapter have been previously published in *The Essentials of Nursing: An Introduction:* Collins & Parker, published by Macmillan Education Limited.

References

Aitken, R.C.B. (1969) Measurement of feelings using visual analogue scales, *Proceeding of The Royal Society of Medicine*, **62**, 1–8.

Benson, H. (1975) *The Relaxation Response*. William Morrow, New York.

Bonica, J.J. (1980) Cancer pain. In Bonica, J.J. (ed.) *Pain*. Raven Press, New York, pp. 335–362.

Bourbinais, F. (1981) Pain assessment: Development of a tool for the nurse and patient, *Journal of Advanced Nursing*, **6**, 277–282.

Bowling, A. (1982) The hospitalisation of death: Should more people die at home? Paper presented at the London Medical Group Symposium, Guy's Hospital.

Bowling, A., and Cartwright, A. (1982) *Life After a Death: A Study of the Elderly Widowed*. Tavistock, London.

Brody, D.S. (1980) The patient's role in clinical decision making. *Annals of Internal Medicine*, **93**, 718–722.

Cartwright, A., Hockey, L., and Anderson, A.B.M. (1973) *Life Before Death*. Routledge & Kegan Paul, London.

Clement Jones, V., Lowry, P.J., Rees, L.H., and Beeser, G.M. (1980a) Met-enkephalin circulates in human plasma, *Nature, London*, **283**, 295–297.

Clement Jones, V., *et al.* (1980b) Increased Beta-endorphin but not Met-enkephalin levels in human cerebral spinal fluid after acupuncture for recurrent pain, *Lancet*, **2**, 946–948.

Connally, G. (1985) New medicine old tricks (biofeedback), *Nursing Times*, September 11, 41–42.

Craig, K.D., and Neidermayer, H. (1974) Autonomic correlates of pain thresholds influenced by sound modeling, *Journal of Personality and Social Psychology*, **29**, 246–252.

Craig, K.D., and Prkachin, K.M. (1978) Social modelling influences on sensory decision theory and psychophysiological indices of pain, *Journal of Personality and Social Psychology*, **36**, (18), 805–815.

Daut, R.L., Cleeland, C.J., and Flanery, R.C. (1983) Development of the Wisconsin Brief Pain Questionnaire to assess pain in cancer and other diseases, *Pain*, **17**, 197–210.

Davitz, L.J., and Davitz, J.R. (1975) How nurses view patient suffering. In *Studies of Nursing Behaviours*. Springer, New York.

De Crosta, T. (1984) Relieving pain: Four non-invasive ways you should know more about, *Nursing Life*, **4**, Part 2, 28–33.

Diggory, G., and Tiffany, R. (1979) The use of Entonox in the relief of pain, *Cancer Nursing*, August, 279–282.

Donovan, M. (1980) Relaxation with guided imagery: A useful technique, *Cancer Nursing*, February, 27–32.

Downie, W.W., Leatham, P.A., Rhine, V.M., Weight, V., Bronco, J.A., and Anderson, J.A. (1978) Studies with pain rating scales, Annals of the rheumatic diseases, *Pain*, **8**, 377–387.

Engel, G.L. (1959) Psychogenic pain and the pain prone patient, *American Journal of Medicine*, **26**, 899–918.

Fraser, F.W. (1978) Persistent post-sympathetic pain treated by connective tissue massage, *Physiotherapy*, **64** (7), 221–212.

Goldscheider, A.C. (1898) *Uber den Schmerz: Gesammette Abhandlungen*, Vol. 1, p. 432, Leipzig.

Goleman, D. (1979) Holographic memory, *Psychology Today*, February, 71–84.

Grant, A.E. (1964) Massage with ice (cryokinetics) in the treatment of painful conditions of the musculoskeletal system, *Archives of Physical Medicine & Rehabilitation*, May, 223–238.

Hackett, T.P. (1971) Pain and prejudice: Why do we doubt that the patient is in pain? *Medical Times*, **99** (2), 130.

Hardy, J.D., Wolff, H.G., and Goodell, H. (1952) *Pain Sensations and Reactions*. Williams & Williams, Baltimore.

Head, H., and Rivers, C. (1920) *Studies in Neurology*. Oxford Medical Publications, Oxford.

Hinton, J.M. (1963) The physical and mental distress of the dying, *Quarterly Journal of Medicine*, **125**, 1–21.

Hockley, J. (1983) An investigation to identify symptoms of distress in the terminally ill patient and his/her family in the general medical ward. Nursing Research Papers, City & Hackney Health District No. 2.

Hunt, J.M., *et al.* (1978) Patients with protracted pain, a survey conducted at The London Hospital, *Journal of Medical Ethics*, **3**, 61–73.

Huskisson, E.C. (1974) Measurement of pain, *Lancet*, **2**, 1127–1131.

Jessell, T.M., and Iverson, L.L. (1977) Opiate analgesics inhibitor substance P release from rat trigeminal nucleus, *Nature*, **268**, 549–551.

Johnson, J.E. (1972) Effects of structuring patients' expectations on the reactions to threatening events, *Nursing Research*, **21**, 499–504.

Johnson, J.E. (1973) Effects of accurate expectations about sensations on the sensory and distress components of pain, *Journal of Personality and Social Psychology*, **27**, 261–275.

Johnson, J.E., and Rice, V.H. (1974) Sensory and distress components of pain: Implications for the study of clinical pain. *Nursing Research*, **23**, 203–209.

Keele, K.D. (1948) The pain chart, *Lancet*, **ii**, 6–8.

Krebs, D.L. (1975) Empathy and altrusion, *Journal of Personality and Social Psychology*, **32** (6), 134–1140.

Lasagna, I.C. (1960) The clinical measurement of pain, *Annals of New York Academy of Science*, **86**, 28–30.

Lewis, G. (1978) The place of pain in human experience, *Journal of Medical Ethics*, **3**, 122–123.

Littlejohns, D.W., and Vere, D.W. (1981) The clinical assessment of analgesic drugs. *British Journal of Clinical Pharmacology*, April 11, 319–332.

Livingston, W.K. (1943) *Pain Mechanisms*. Macmillan, New York.

Loeser, J.D. (1980) Low back pain. *Res. Publ. Assoc. Nerv. Ment. Dis.*, **58**, 363–377.

Lunt, B. (1980) Terminal cancer care: Specialist services available in Great Britain. University of Southampton in conjunction with Wessex Regional Cancer Organisation.

Maclean, R.A. (1975) *Triune Concept of Brain and Behaviour*. Toronto Press, Toronto, pp. 6–60.

Marks, R.M., and Sachar, E.J. (1973) Undertreatment of medical inpatients with narcotic analgesics, *Ann. Intern. Med.*, **78**, 173–181.

Mayer, D.J., and Price, D.D. (1977) Raf ii, 4. *Brain Research*, **121**, 368–372.

Maxwell, J. (1978) Sensitivity and accuracy of The visual Analogue Scales. A psycho-physical classroom experiment, *British Journal of Pharmacology*, **6**, 15–24.

McCaffery, M. (1979a) *Nursing the Patient in Pain*. Adapted for the UK by Beatrice Sofaer. Harper & Row, London.

McCaffery, M. (1979b) *Nursing Management of the Patient with Pain.* Lippincott, Philadelphia.

McGuire, D.B. (1984) The measurement of clinical pain, *Nursing Research*, **33** (3), 152–156.

Melzack, R. (1975) The McGill Pain Questionnaire: Major properties and scoring methods, *Pain*, **1**, 277–299.

Melzack, R. and Denis, S.G. (1978) Pain-signalling in the dorsal and ventral spinal cord. *Pain*, **4** (2), 97–132.

Melzack, R., and Torgerson, W.J. (1971) On the language of pain, *Anaesthesiology*, **34**, 50–59.

Melzack, R., and Wall, P.D. (1965) Pain mechanisms: A new theory, *Int. Science*, **150**, 971–9.

Melzack, R., and Wall, P.D. (1982) *The Challenge of Pain.* Penguin, Harmondsworth.

Ostrowski, M.B. (1977) Transcutaneous nerve stimulation for relief of pain in advanced malignant disease. *Nursing Times*, August 11, 1233–1238.

Parkes, C.M. (1978) Home or hospital? Patterns of care for the terminally ill cancer patient as seen by surviving spouses, *Journal of the Royal College of General Practitioners*, **28**, 19–30.

Pilowsky, I., and Bond, M.R. (1969) Pain and its management in malignant disease *Psychosomatic Medicine*, **31**, 400–404.

Pomeranz, B., and Chui, D. (1976) Naloxone blockade of acupuncture analgesia: Endorphin implicated, *Life Sci.*, **19**, 1757–1762.

Raiman, J.A. (1986a) Pain relief, a two-way process. *Nursing Times*, **82** (15), 24–28.

Raiman, J.A. (1986b) Monitoring pain at home, *Journal of District Nursing*, **4** (11), 4–6.

Raiman, J.A. (1986c) Towards understanding pain, and planning for relief, *Nursing*, **3** (11), 411–423.

Reading, A.E. (1980) A comparison of pain rating scales, *Journal of Psychosomatic Research*, **24**, 119–124.

Scott, J., and Huskisson, E.C. (1976) Graphic representation of pain, *Pain*, **2**, 175–184.

Sternbach, R., and Tursky, B. (1965) Ethnic differences among housewives in psychophysical and skin potential responses to electric shock, *Psychophysiology*, **1**, 241–246.

Szasz, T.T., and Hollender, M.H. (1956) A contribution to the philosophy of medicine: The basic models of the doctor–patient relationship. *Annals of Internal Medicine*, **97**, 585–592.

Tournier, P. (1957) *The Meaning of Persons.* S.C.M., London, p. 137.

Twycross, R.G. (1976) Diseases of the central nervous system. Relief of terminal pain. *British Medical Journal*, **4**, (5990), 212–214.

Twycross, R.G., and Fairfield, S. (1982) Pain in far-advanced cancer, *Pain*, **14**, 303–310.

Van Ree, J.M., De Wied, D., Bradbury, A.F., Hulme, E.C., Smyth, D.G., and Snell, C.R. (1976) *Nature*, **264**, 792–794.

Wall, P.D., and Sweet, W.H. (1967) *Science*, **155**, 108.

Wallace, H. and Benson, H. (1972) The psychology of meditation, *Scientific American*, **226**, 85–90.

Weisenberg, M. (1977) *Psychol. Bulletin*, **4**, 1008–1044.

Woodford, J.M., and Merskey, H. (1972) Some relationships between subjective measures of pain, *Journal of Psychosomatic Research*, **16**, 173–178.

Zborowski, M. (1969) *People in Pain.* Jossey Bass, San Francisco.

Nursing Issues and Research in Terminal Care
Edited by J. Wilson-Barnett and J. Raiman
© 1988 John Wiley & Sons Ltd.

CHAPTER 8

Complementary Therapies as Nursing Interventions

SALLY SIMS

Chapter Contents

This chapter discusses the role of complementary therapies as nursing interventions in terminal care. In particular it reviews relevant research on the benefits of relaxation training, touch, massage and music therapy in patient care and suggests that these techniques have immediate practical application in the terminal care setting since they are non-invasive, may enhance patient comfort and can be safely carried out by nurses following minimal instruction. Nurses are in an excellent position to be able to evaluate such therapies for the potential benefits they may have for patients; directions for future research are therefore outlined at the end of each section.

Introduction

Over the past 20 years there has been a growing interest in 'complementary' or 'unorthodox' approaches to care by both lay persons and health professionals alike. Complementary care is a term which is frequently adopted in preference to 'alternative medicine' because it is widely believed that techniques such as relaxation training and acupuncture should complement, rather than provide an alternative to, traditional medical treatments (Inglis and West, 1983). It is also more appropriate to refer to complementary 'care' rather than 'medicine', since the majority of techniques remain largely independent of and unaccepted by conventional medicine.

Complementary approaches to care are often discussed under the collective term 'holistic therapies'. Complementary care may or may not be holistic. Holism refers to a principle of care rather than to specific therapies or techniques. Holism embraces four main principles: responding to the person as a whole in his environment, seeing the individual as a combination of mind, body and spirit; willingness to use a wide range of interventions including both orthodox and complementary therapies; encouraging the patient's self-responsibility; and recognizing the importance of the practitioner's own health (British Holistic Medical Association, 1987). Traditional medicine has been criticized for treating specific parts of the body rather than considering the total person (Green, Green and Walter, 1970); however, recognition of the principles of holism has grown in recent years, as evidenced by the shift towards individualized patient care and the growth of the hospice movement, which stresses the importance of caring for the total person (Saunders, 1980). Interest in complementary therapies has also grown in recent years. This has been interpreted by some as pointing to the failure of medicine to satisfy the public's health care needs (Inglis and West, 1983). In response to this the medical profession is quick to point out that there is little evidence to substantiate the claimed effects of the majority of complementary therapies (*Lancet*, 1983). As very few empirical studies have been carried out in this area, for the most part only hypotheses can be offered. In spite of this, it would appear shortsighted to deny the patient access to therapies which, although poorly substantiated as yet, may provide some benefit for the patient. Nurses are in an excellent position to be able to incorporate into patient care complementary therapies which may enhance physical and psychological comfort and to systematically evaluate the outcomes. When cure is no longer possible and the emphasis of treatment shifts to comfort, care and symptom control, complementary therapies may be particularly beneficial. It should not be forgotten, however, that terminally ill patients are potentially vulnerable. They may seek complementary therapies for a possible cure and be unable to distinguish between genuine practitioners and the charismatic salesman. In light of the current interest in complementary care by both lay and professional persons, nurses must be aware of the uses and limitations of such techniques and must be prepared to communicate caution, as well as alerting patients to the possible benefits.

There are at least 30 different techniques which are commonly considered under the heading of complementary care (see Table 1). Only a small number of these techniques have immediate practical

Table 1. Therapies and techniques commonly included under the heading of complementary care

Acupunture	Kirlean photography
Aikido	Massage
Alexander technique	Meditation
Aromatherapy	Music therapy
Autogenic training	Naturopathy
Bach remedies	Osteopathy
Biochemics	Reflexology
Biofeedback	Relaxation techniques
Chiropractic	Rolfing
Colour therapy	Shiatsu
Guided imagery	Sound therapy
Herbal medicine	Spiritual healing
Homeopathy	Tai Chi
Hydrotherapy	Therapeutic touch
	Yoga

application in nursing in terms of being non-invasive, potentially comfort-promoting and requiring little additional instruction. They include:

— Relaxation techniques
— Touch and massage
— Music therapy

Although these techniques have received support in the nursing literature, relatively few studies have been carried out by nurses to evaluate their use in nursing in general and in the terminal care setting in particular. Relevant nursing studies in each of the above areas will therefore be reviewed in order to highlight the practice implications for terminal nursing care and directions for future research.

Relaxation Techniques

The potential benefit of relaxation training has generated widespread interest in both the lay and professional literature, particularly in the area of stress management. The value of relaxation techniques aimed at reducing the level of physiological arousal and subjective distress may be particularly great for patients who are facing death. Terminal illness places considerable physiological and psychological demands on the patient and may evoke significant emotional distress (see Chapter

5, Coping with Dying). Relaxation training can assist an individual to control the body's response to stress and therefore reduce the severity of the stress reaction (Benson, 1975).

Definitions

Relaxation refers to a state at the lower end of a continuum of arousal. The relaxation response is a hypothalamic response which leads to a reduction in the activity of the sympathetic nervous system and a concomitant decrease in oxygen consumption, decreased muscle tone, heart rate, respiratory rate and body metabolism (Benson, 1975). The relaxation response is also accompanied by decreased anxiety (Goldfried and Trier, 1974). Anxiety and muscular relaxation produce opposing physiological effects and cannot exist together. The relaxation response in man, therefore, consists of changes opposite to those of the flight or fight, or stress response (Benson, Beary and Carol, 1974).

Benson, Beary and Carol (1974) state that four basic elements are usually necessary to elicit the relaxation response:

— A constant stimulus such as a word, sound, phrase or tactile stimulus which facilitates a shift away from externally orientated thought.
— A passive attitude and the ability to disregard distracting thoughts and redirect them towards the technique
— Decreased muscle tone
— A quiet environment

There are a number of different relaxation techniques which may elicit the relaxation response, including transcendental meditation, yoga, hypnosis, biofeedback, progressive muscle relaxation, guided imagery and deep rhythmical breathing. The two techniques which have received most attention in the nursing literature are progressive muscle relaxation and guided imagery.

Progressive muscle relaxation was originally introduced by Jacobsen in the 1920s. Although a number of different variations of Jacobsen's technique have evolved, the underlying principle remains the same. By progressively tensing and relaxing different muscle groups, the subject is taught to induce low levels of tension in the major muscles and to discriminate between feelings experienced when the muscle is tense compared with relaxed (Snyder, 1985). Many progressive muscle relaxation techniques also require the individual to focus on breathing rhythmically and deeply and some incorporate guided imagery (visualization), a technique which involves focusing on pleasant images in the imagination in order to induce relaxation (Sodergren, 1985).

Evaluation of Progressive Muscle Relaxation and Guided Imagery in Nursing

Progressive muscle relaxation

Relaxation training has been used to help patients with a number of different conditions. In the main the focus has been on the reduction of anxiety (Goldfried and Trier, 1974), hypertension (Barr-Taylor *et al.*, 1977), tension headaches (Cox, Freundlich and Meyer, 1978), insomnia (Weil and Goldfried, 1973) and alleviating the side-effects of chemotherapy (Burish and Lyles, 1981). The majority of papers have been published in the psychology, psychiatry, medical and behavioural science journals. Since the late 1970s, however, an increasing number of papers on the use of relaxation techniques have appeared in the nursing literature. The following therapeutic effects of progressive muscle relaxation have been examined by nurses:

— *Pain reduction*
Postoperative pain (Flaherty and Fitzpatrick, 1978; Wells, 1982)
— *Anxiety reduction*
Frequency of intake of PRN tranquillizers (Tamez *et al.*, 1978)
Relief of anxiety associated with chemotherapy and clinic visits (Moore and Altmaier, 1981)
— *Symptom distress reduction*
Relief of nausea, vomiting and anxiety associated with chemotherapy (Cotanch, 1983)

Flaherty and Fitzpatrick (1978) examined the effects of teaching progressive muscle relaxation preoperatively to 42 general surgical patients, on perceived comfort when getting out of bed following surgery. They found a significant difference in analgesia, incisional pain, bodily distress and respirations in patients who had received relaxation training compared with the control group. Differences in heart rate and blood pressure were not significant. In a two-group pre- and post-test experimental design, Wells (1982) set out to determine whether there was a significant difference in muscle tension and postoperative pain in six patients who had received relaxation training prior to cholecystectomy compared with six patients who had received standard preoperative preparation. Wells (1982) found that relaxation training appeared to reduce the psychological discomfort of pain but had no measurable effects on abdominal muscle tension. Unlike Flaherty and Fitzpatrick (1978), no differences in the amount of analgesics used were found.

As these studies focused on the effects of progressive muscle relaxation on acute pain, further studies are needed to determine whether progressive muscle relaxation can help to alleviate the chronic pain experienced in terminal illness. The effectiveness of relaxation techniques in modifying the perception can be explained in terms of the gate control theory of Melzack and Wall (1965). Focusing on relaxing muscles may serve as a distraction from the pain stimulus, closing the gating mechanism to pain impulses. In addition, anxiety is reduced, modifying pain perception, and the relaxation of muscular tension means that the cycle of pain–spasm–pain is interrupted. Although it is not yet clear exactly how relaxation training lowers anxiety, Goldfried and Trier (1974) suggest there is little doubt that it does. Some evidence is accumulating to substantiate this claim. Moore and Altmaier (1981) found that four out of seven patients reported reduced anxiety associated with clinic visits and chemotherapy following relaxation training and Cotanch (1983) also reports that relaxation may be beneficial in reducing the anxiety, nausea and vomiting associated with chemotherapy. Nine out of twelve patients in her nursing research study reported some benefit following relaxation training. Neither of these studies included a control group, however. Further research is needed to explore the potential benefits of progressive muscle relaxation for symptom distress and anxiety in different patient groups including the terminally ill.

Progressive muscle relaxation is generally believed to have few if any negative side-effects; however, some precautions have been suggested. Progressive muscle relaxation may be very tiring for the weak since a sustained effort is required to elicit the response and the subject may have difficulty acquiring the skill (Kaempfer, 1982). Patients with dyspnoea may find it difficult to focus on their breathing (Donovan, 1980) and total relaxation may produce a hypotensive state (Synder, 1985). Benson, Beary and Carol (1974) caution that if the relaxation response is elicited more than two periods of 20–30 minutes daily, some may experience withdrawal from life and symptoms ranging from insomnia to hallucinations.

Guided imagery

There is a lack of nursing research on the use of guided imagery in nursing. McCaffery (1979) suggests that imagery may be used to assist patients to alleviate pain through eliciting relaxation and focusing on stimuli other than the pain, although no research is given in support of this. Other hypothesized benefits include alleviation of hopelessness (Smith, 1982), facilitating relaxation with progressive muscle relaxation (Donovan, 1980) and the exploration of repressed ideas (Sodergren, 1985). The lack of controlled studies concerning the effects of imagery on specific outcomes means that nurses must rely on practical experience to suggest possible areas of benefit. Caution is best taken in interpreting images which are elicited by the patient and appropriate psychological care is needed in response to any emotions which are evoked.

Directions for Future Research

Numerous studies have been carried out outside of nursing to determine the effects of relaxation and relaxation training. By comparison, few studies have been carried out by nurses to evaluate the benefits of relaxation techniques such as progressive muscle relaxation and guided imagery, although the nursing literature acknowledges that they may be beneficial for some patients. Further research is needed across all patient groups and in particular with terminally ill patients. Possible topics for further research in the terminal care setting include studies:

— To identify the ways in which relaxation training may be beneficial for terminally ill patients
— To determine the effects of relaxation training on specific outcomes such as chronic pain, anxiety and symptom distress in terminally ill patients
— To identify which relaxation techniques are most suitable for terminally ill patients
— To determine the characteristics of patients who may benefit from relaxation training and those who may not
— To determine whether teaching relaxation techniques to terminally ill patients can enhance perceived coping ability.

Studies could also be extended to include an evaluation of the benefits of relaxation training for the carers of terminally ill patients, as working with the terminally ill has been shown to be a stressful area of care (Benoliel, 1983).

Touch and Massage

Over the centuries touch has played an important part in many of the different complementary therapies. More recently research has started to accumulate and evidence suggests that touch and massage may facilitate health and well-being.

Definitions

Touch in this context is used to refer to three different types of touch: expressive touch, which is purposeful physical contact with the patient, excluding touching that occurs while performing other tasks (Watson, 1975), therapeutic touch, which is a form of healing touch involving the transference of energy (Krieger, 1979), and massage. Massage is a systematic form of touch and comprises different movements and sequences ranging from a gentle back rub to the art practised by professional therapists. Massage therapy involves the manipulation of the soft tissues for therapeutic purposes (Beard and Wood, 1964) but as a generic term includes specific techniques such as slow stroke back massage, shiatsu and reflexology. Slow stroke back massage is a slow, rhythmic back massage comprised of gentle strokes performed with both hands over the back (Sims, 1986). Shiatsu is a pressure form of massage often used in conjunction with traditional massage strokes (Vega, 1975), and reflexology is a specific massage of the feet and hands based on the assumption that the entire body is reflected there (Zeller-Dobbs, 1985).

Evaluation of Touch and Massage in Nursing

Expressive touch

Touch is one of the first senses to develop and is a fundamental way of communicating (Montagu, 1978). The need and desire to communicate with others is basic to the nature of man. Through purposeful, expressive touch, the nurse may be able to demonstrate sensitivity and both permit and facilitate the expression of feelings. Nursing research indicates that purposeful touch is recognized and appreciated by patients. In her study of the effects of touching the arm of seriously ill patients throughout a conversation, McCorkle (1974) found that the patients' responses were more positive and demonstrated less tension behaviour than the non-touch group. In addition, the patients interacted more with the nurses and were more attentive. Knable (1981) reports positive psychological responses to purposefully holding the hands of critically ill patients in an intensive care unit. Knable (1981) noted that after the nurses had terminated the interaction the patients sometimes reinitiated the handholding. Both appropriate timing and serious intent were found to be necessary in order for handholding to be therapeutic.

The patient who is terminally ill may find purposeful expressive touch particularly beneficial. A caring sympathetic touch may communicate security, reawaken an individual's remaining perceptual capacity, facilitate communication and prevent isolation and social withdrawal. According to Kubler Ross (1970), a gentle pressure on the hand is one of the most meaningful communications that a nurse can have with a dying patient. However, the use of expressive touch as an intervention for facilitating communication, comforting and orientating dying patients requires further study. In planning and providing touching measures, the nurse must take into consideration the patient's mental, physical and sociocultural status as well as her own feelings about touch. These factors are complex and influence whether or not touch is accepted. De Augustinis, Isani and Kumler (1963) and De Wever (1977) have found that correct understanding of the meaning of the nurse's touch cannot always be assumed.

Therapeutic touch

Therapeutic touch is the enhancement of patient wellbeing and healing through touch based on the concept of energy transference. Therapeutic touch has received much attention in recent years, particularly in the American nursing literature, and was originally described by Krieger in the 1970s. A declaration of religious faith is not necessary in order for therapeutic touch to be effective, and although bodily contact may be made, the hands are usually held just above the subject's body · (Krieger, 1981). Therapeutic touch is carried out on the premise that excess energy from the helping person can be transferred to the patient in order to repattern his lowered energy pattern, which is considered to be the basis of all ill-health. The transfer of energy is intentional and comes about when the helper is in a state of 'healing meditation' focusing all thoughts, actions and energies on the patient's needs (Krieger, 1979).

Krieger (1979) and others report that therapeutic touch may have a number of beneficial effects for the patient. Krieger (1979) states that it may induce relaxation and help to alleviate pain as well as other symptoms such as nausa, dyspnoea and tachycardia. Nursing studies by Heidt (1981) and Quinn (1984) suggest that therapeutic touch may also lead to a reduction in the anxiety levels of hospitalized patients.

Although therapeutic touch may be beneficial for certain patients, caution is required in the interpretation of these results since tools which can measure interactions in terms of energy transference are lacking. In the case of the terminally ill patient, care must be taken to ensure that the patient interprets the meaning of the touch accurately in order to avoid instilling false hopes of cure.

Massage

Massage has been used since the earliest of times in the treatment of a variety of conditions. The effects of massage are varied and depend upon the strokes being used and the pressure being exerted. Massage effects can be broadly classified as being psychological, reflex and mechanical (Table 2).

A number of authors have described how nurses in the USA (Temple, 1967; Hardy, 1975; Michelsen, 1978) and in the UK (Holmes, 1986) have incorporated massage into patient care in order to promote sleep, relieve muscle tension and ease aching muscles. Few nursing research studies have been carried out, however, to evaluate the use of massage in patient care or to explore the potential benefits massage may have for patients. To date, nursing studies have focused on the effects of massage in three main areas:

— *Relaxation*
Effects of back rub on autonomic function (Kaufmann, 1964)
Psychophysiological effects of slow stroke back massage (Longworth, 1982)
— *Comfort levels*
Effects of touch and massage during labour (Lorensen, 1983)

— *Perceived well-being*
Patients with inflammatory bowel disease (Joachim, 1983)
Female cancer patients receiving radiotherapy (Sims, 1986)

Kaufmann (1964) studied the autonomic responses of eighteen male and eighteen female medical patients following a back rub, compared with a control intervention of lying down. Galvanic skin response, systolic blood pressure, pulse rate and the patient's perception of the intervention were recorded. Kaufmann's (1964) findings were inconclusive but the rather invasive recording procedure may have interfered with the effect of the massage. She was able to state,

Table 2. Summary of massage effects

Psychological	Reflex	Mechanical
Reduction of anxiety	Vasodilation of blood vessels (Scull, 1945)	Emptying of lymphatics Increased circulation and decreased absorption of toxic substances (Scull, 1945)
Facilitation of positive relationships and disclosure of concerns (Woody, 1980)	Stimulation or sedation of CNS (Beard and Wood, 1964)	Increased diuresis and increased peristalsis (following abdominal massage) (Beard and Wood, 1964)
	Reduction of muscle tension and relaxation of muscles from spasm (Scull, 1945)	
	Relief from pain due to reduction of muscle tension and release of endogenous opiates (De Crosta, 1984)	Increased skin temperature (Beard and Wood, 1964)
	Increased trunk flexibility (Nordshow and Bierman, 1962)	

however, that the verbal responses were 'almost entirely of a strongly positive nature'. Longworth (1982) successfully demonstrated a significant decrease in blood pressure, pulse rate and anxiety following a slow stroke back massage on 32 healthy females. However, as only a convenience sample of healthy subjects and no control group were used, generalizations from the results cannot be made.

Lorensen (1983) found that touch during labour, including a gentle back rub, was perceived as helpful by twelve primigravidae in relieving the discomfort of childbirth. This study was small and lacked randomization. Joachim (1983) carried out a small pilot study to determine the effects of deep abdominal breathing and massage on the wellbeing of fifteen patients with inflammatory bowel disease. All of the patients reported that the massage rather than the deep abdominal breathing made them feel more relaxed. The poor research design and lack of control group severely limits the significance of these findings. In another small pilot study, Sims (1986) set out to determine the effects of slow stroke back massage on the perceived wellbeing of six female patients receiving radiotherapy for breast cancer. Sims (1986) found that overall the patients reported less symptom distress, higher degrees of tranquillity and vitality and less tension and tiredness following slow stroke back massage, compared with a control intervention of lying down. In addition, patients' comments following the massage were of a positive nature. However, the small scale of the study and lack of statistically significant findings limits the extent to which the findings can be generalized.

It has been suggested that the need for touch increases in times of stress (Barnett, 1972). It is therefore appropriate that nurses continue to evaluate how different touching techniques such as massage may be used in stress-related situations. Nurses in the terminal care setting are in an ideal position to be able to offer gentle massage and systematically evaluate the outcome. Massage should always be given thoughtfully and with due consideration of any underlying pathology. Patients who have thrombophlebitis should not be given calf massage because of the risk of emboli formation (Knapp, 1971) and massage is also contraindicated where there is a risk of spreading infection throughout the tissues (e.g. cellulitis) or of spreading infection by contact (e.g. boils) (Knapp, 1971). It has been suggested that massage may promote tumour extension and metastases (Knapp, 1971). When massaging cancer patients gentle strokes are therefore preferable and care must be taken to ensure that no disease exists in the skin or subcutaneous tissues at the site of massage application.

Shiatsu and reflexology

Shiatsu and reflexology have stimulated some interest in the nursing literature. It has been suggested that Shiatsu (Vega, 1975; Box, 1984) and reflexology (Lett, 1983; Zeller-Dobbs, 1985) should be incorporated into patient care. Research findings to support these claims are, however, lacking.

Shiatsu involves the application of pressure at particular points along the body's main energy channels or meridians in order to balance the body's energy flow. The points used are similar to those used in acupuncture. Pressure may be applied by the fingers, forearms, elbows, palms, soles of the feet and toes (Box, 1984). Pressure is varied according to the malady being treated and similar physiological effects to massage and acupuncture are claimed (Vega, 1975). Although a number of practitioners claim clinical success with Shiatsu, the value of Shiatsu in nursing needs further enquiry.

Reflexology refers to the massage of specific reflex zones on the hands and feet which represent particular parts of the body (Lett, 1983). Zeller-Dobbs (1985) describes how she has used reflexology with terminally ill cancer patients to decrease pain, provide relaxation, encourage physical contact and diminish isolation, although no research is given in support of this. Zeller-Dobbs (1985) also reports that where relatives have been taught to give reflexology, the relative often benefits as much as the patient. Reflexology may provide a way of helping terminally ill patients feel more supported and may enhance well-being; however, further research is necessary to substantiate these claims.

Directions for Future Research

Although touch is widely used in nursing, relatively few studies have been carried out to determine the potential benefits purposeful touch and specific touching techniques such as massage, Shiatsu and reflexology may have for patients. Further studies are needed to explore and provide a more scientific basis for the use of touch and massage techniques in nursing across all patient groups. In the terminal care setting directions for future research include studies:

— To determine the types of purposeful touch terminally ill patients perceive as beneficial
— To determine whether terminally ill patients have greater need for touch than other patients
— To determine the benefits of purposeful touch for specific outcomes such as pain, anxiety, loneliness
— To determine the effects of expressive touch *versus* therapeutic touch
— To determine the effect of different massage techniques including slow stroke back massage, Shiatsu and reflexology on specific patient outcomes and to compare and contrast the results.

Music Therapy

Throughout history music has been used in a variety of different ways for therapeutic purposes. Alvin (1966) provides a comprehensive account of the history of the use of music as therapy. Ideally the most qualified person to provide music as an intervention in patient care is a music therapist, who has received specialized training based on a thorough knowledge of music, the behavioural sciences and accepted therapeutic approaches. However, as Cook (1981) points out, most clinical areas are not staffed with music therapists. This need not prevent the use of music in patient care for, as Munro and Mount (1978) state, 'Any motivated person irrespective of training may effectively use music in ministering to the sick'. By being aware of the potential uses of music, nurses with some musical knowledge can judiciously incorporate its use into many clinical situations. Indeed, the increasing number of articles which have appeared in the nursing literature on this subject indicates that nurses may be awakening to the potential benefits of integrating music into patient care (Parriott, 1969; Gilbert, 1977; Herth, 1978; Loscin, 1981; Cook, 1981; Snyder, 1985). Dentists have for some time been the leading proponents of music, using it to promote relaxation and pain control in their patients (Jacobsen, 1956).

Definition

Music therapy is the controlled use of music in the treatment, rehabilitation, education and learning of children and adults suffering from physical, mental or emotional disorder (Alvin, 1966). The characteristics of the music and the effect it produces depend upon the different elements of the sound and the relationship between them. Alvin (1966) describes five elements of music:

— Frequency (pitch)
— Intensity
— Tone colour (timbre)
— Interval (distance between two notes)
— Duration and rhythm

  Music therapy can take many forms (Sachett and Fitzgerald, 1980), including:

— Creative music, e.g. informal group singing, playing an instrument, either individually or in a group
— Music appreciation, e.g. listening to live or taped music either individually or in a group
— Music discussion, e.g. discussing the feelings which a certain piece of music is trying to portray

— Carrying out other activities to music, e.g. drawing or painting. Refer to Johnson and Berendt (1986) for the value of art therapy in nursing.

Evaluation of Music Therapy in Nursing

Gilbert (1977) suggests that music therapy offers a rich, largely untapped potential for use with terminally ill patients and their relatives. Based on ten years' clinical experience with music therapy at the Royal Victoria Hospital in Montreal, Munro and Mount (1978) propose the following potential benefits of music therapy for patients receiving palliative care, although only case reports are given in support of these claims.

Physical
— Relaxation
— Pain relief through relieving anxiety and depression
— Facilitating physical exercise

Psychological
— Altering mood, reducing anxiety
— Reinforcing identity and self-concept
— Non-verbal means of communication
— Stimulating recall of past events
— Reinforcing reality or expressing fantasy

Social
— Socially acceptable means of self-expression
— Decreased isolation
— Providing a link with the patient's life before illness
— Providing an opportunity for group participation (the dynamics of the group may be just as important as the actual therapy (Gilbert, 1977)

Spiritual
— Providing a means for expressing spirituality and emotions

Although music therapy would appear to have considerable potential for nursing and terminal care there is a lack of systematic study in all care settings. The following authors provide anecdotal evidence of the benefit of music as a nursing intervention. Herth (1978) used music to assist postsurgical patients in getting out of bed. She encouraged patients to listen to their favourite music for about five minutes prior to getting out of bed and found that feelings of lightheadedness and fainting were reduced. Munro and Mount (1978) present several patient case studies to highlight the benefits of music in palliative care. In one case the combination of guided imagery and music was so effective that in the last days of life analgesics could be discontinued completely.

In an unpublished nursing thesis, Cook (1981) used soothing music with oncology patients who were receiving radiotherapy. The experimental group had significantly lower anxiety scores ten days into the treatment than the control group. The patients reported that the music made the treatment appear shorter, reduced the noise level of the environment and made the treatment less stressful. In another nursing study, Loscin (1981) investigated the effects of music on postoperative pain. The patient's preferred choice of music was played for fifteen minutes every two hours for the first 48 hours after surgery. It was found that patients in the experimental group had lower musculoskeletal and verbal pain scores, lower blood pressure and pulse rates than patients in the control group. Loscin (1981) concluded that music decreases the overt pain reaction of patients during the first 48 hours postoperatively.

Cook (1981) cautions against generalizing about the effects of music since individuals react differently to the same music. It is important to assess the particular needs of each patient and to introduce music thoughtfully into patient care, since patients may have little defence against the impact of music. Snyder (1985) suggests that playing music without first assessing the likes and dislikes of a patient could be harmful. Selecting and organizing music therapy may be time-consuming. Thought needs to be given to the type of music used, when to use it and how. Some knowledge of music is therefore advantageous. Just turning on the radio does not constitute music therapy. Although music is a readily available intervention, the cost of instruments may be prohibitive and a room which is sufficiently soundproofed, so as to not disturb others, may be required.

Directions for Future Research

Although used little by nurses in the past, music may have a wide variety of applications in patient care. If used judiciously, music has the potential of becoming a valuable nursing intervention. Nurses should work closely with music therapists to explore the potential benefits of music for different patient groups. In the terminal care setting directions for future research include studies:

— To determine which types of music therapy are most beneficial in a terminal care setting
— To determine the effects of different types of music on specific outcomes such as pain and anxiety
— To explore the benefits of music together with other creative therapies such as art or poetry for the patient who is terminally ill

Conclusion

As recently as 20 years ago it seemed unlikely that complementary therapies, which were often considered to be old-fashioned, outmoded forms of treatment practised by 'quacks', would survive. Significant interest in complementary care has been revived so that today the proportion of people who use complementary therapies has increased considerably. The medical profession has also begun to take complementary therapies more seriously and has identified the need to carry out research projects designed to compare conventional with unconventional forms of treatment (*Lancet*, 1983). Complementary care has aroused significant interest among nurses, who have addressed its implications for nursing at a number of international conferences. Nurses have been slow, however, to evaluate specific techniques for the potential benefits they may have for patients. It may well be that the scepticism of medical (and nursing) colleagues has hindered this process. Personal experience attests to the difficulties in obtaining medical support for therapies such as slow stroke back massage, which may be perceived as 'bizarre' or 'way out'. In the terminal care setting, where the emphasis is on symptom control and comfort care rather than medical treatment and cure, it may be easier for nurses to examine complementary care techniques which are non-invasive and carry little risk but which may enhance patients' physical and psychological wellbeing. It is hoped that nurses in the terminal care setting will take up this challenge.

References

Alvin, J. (1966) *Music Therapy*. John Clare Books, London.
Barnett, K. (1972) A theoretical construct of the concepts of touch as they relate to nursing. *Nursing Research*, **21** (2), 102–109.

Barr-Taylor, C., Farquhar, J., Nelson, E., and Agras, S. (1977) Relaxation therapy and high blood pressure, *Arch. Gen. Psychiatry*, **34**, 339–342.

Beard, G., and Wood, G. (1964) *Massage Principles and Techniques*. W.B. Saunders, Philadelphia and London.

Benoliel, J.O. (1983) Nursing research on death, dying and terminal illness development, present State and prospects, *Annual Review of Nursing Research*, Vol. 1, Chapter 5, pp. 101–130.

Benson, H. (1975) *The Relaxation Response*. William Morrow, New York.

Benson, H., Beary, J., and Carol, M. (1974) The relaxation response, *Psychiatry*, **37**, 37–47.

Box, D. (1984) Made in Japan. Holistic health 3, *Nursing Times*, April 25, 39–40.

British Holistic Medical Association (1987) In *Lampada Spring* (II). Royal College of Nursing, London, 46.

Burish, T., and Lyles, J. (1981) Effectiveness of relaxation training in reducing adverse reactions to cancer chemotherapy, *Journal of Behavioural Medicine*, **4** (1), 65–78.

Cook, J.D. (1981) The therapeutic use of music: A literature review, *Nursing Forum*, **XX** (3), 252–266.

Cotanch, P. (1983) Relaxation training for control of nausea and vomiting in patients receiving chemotherapy, *Cancer Nursing*, **4**(6), 277–283.

Cox, D., Freundlich, A., and Meyer, R. (1978) Differential effectiveness of electromyograph feedback, verbal relaxation instructions and medication placebo with tension headaches, *Journal of Consulting and Clinical Psychology*, **43**, 892–898.

De Augustinis, J., Isani, R., and Kumler, F. (1963) Ward study. The meaning of touch in interpersonal communication. In Bard, S., and Marshall, M. (eds) *Some Clinical Approaches to Psychiatric Nursing*. Macmillan, New York.

De Crosta, T. (1984) Reviewing pain: Four non invasive ways you should know more about, *Nursing Life* **2** (4), 28–33.

De Wever, M. (1977) Nursing home patients' perception of nurses' affective touching, *Journal of Psychology*, **96**, 163–171.

Donovan, M. (1980) Relaxation with guided imagery: A useful technique, *Cancer Nursing* **3** (1), 27–32.

Flaherty, G., and Fitzpatrick, J. (1978) Relaxation technique to increase comfort levels of post operative patients: A preliminary study, *Nursing Research*, **27**, 352–355.

Gilbert, J. (1977) Music therapy perspectives on death and dying, *Journal of Music Therapy*, **XIV** (4), 165–171.

Goldfried, M., and Trier, C. (1974) Effectiveness of relaxation as an actve coping skill, *Journal of Abnormal Psychology*, **83** (4), 348–355.

Green, E., Green, A., and Walter, S. (1970) Voluntary control of internal states: psychological and physiological, *Journal of Transpersonal Psychology*, **2** (1), 1–26.

Hardy, J. (1975) The importance of touch, *Journal of Practical Nursing*, **25** (6), 26–27.

Heidt, P. (1981) Effect of therapeutic touch on anxiety level of hospitalized patients, *Nursing Research*, **30** (1), 32–37.

Herth, K. (1978) The therapeutic use of music, *Supervisor Nurse*, **9**, 22–23.

Holmes, P. (1986) Fringe benefits, *Nursing Times*, **82** (22), 20–22.

Inglis, B., and West, R. (1983) *The Alternative Health Guide*. Michael Joseph, London.

Jacobsen, H.C. (1956) The effects of sedative music on the tension, anxiety and pain during the dental procedures, *Bulletin of the National Academy of Music Therapy*, **3**, 9.

Joachim, G. (1983) The effects of two stress management techniques on feelings of well-being in patients with inflammatory bowel disease, *Nurs. Pap.*, **15** (4), 5–18.

Johnson, J., and Berendt, A. (1986) Art and flowers, drawing out the patients' best, *American Journal of Nursing*, February, 164–166.

Kaempfer, S. (1982) Relaxation training reconsidered, *Oncology Nursing Forum*, **2** (9), 15–18.

Kaufmann, M. (1964) Autonomic responses as related to nursing comfort measures, *Nursing Research*, **13** (1), 45–55.

Knable, J. (1981) Handholding: One means of transcending barriers of communication, *Heart and Lung*, **10** (6), 1106–1110.

Knapp, M. (1971) In Krusen, F. *Handbook of Physical Medicine and Rehabilitation*, 2nd edn. W.B. Saunders, London, Chapter 15.

Krieger, D. (1979) Therapeutic touch searching for evidence of physiological change, *American Journal of Nursing*, April, 660–662.

Krieger, D. (1981) *Foundations for Holistic Health Nursing. The Renaissance Nurse*, J.B. Lippincott, Philadelphia.

Kubler Ross, E. (1970) *On Death and Dying*. Tavistock, London.

Lancet (1983) Editorial. Alternative medicine is no alternative, *Lancet*, October 1, 773–774.

Lett, A. (1983) Putting their best feet forward, *Nursing Times*, August 17, 49–51.

Longworth, J. (1982) Psychophysiological effects of slow stroke back massage in normotensive females, *Advances in Nursing Science*, July, 44–61.

Lorensen, M. (1983) Effects of touch in patients during a crisis situation in hospital. In Wilson Barnett, J. (ed.) *Nursing Research: Ten Studies in Patient Care*. Wiley, Chichester, pp. 179–192.

Loscin, R.A. (1981) The effect of music on the pain of selected post operative patients, *Journal of Advanced Nursing*, **6**, 19–25.

McCaffery, M. (1979) *Nursing Management of the Patient with Pain*. J.B. Lippincott, Philadelphia.

McCorkle, R. (1974) Effects of touch on seriously ill patients, *Nursing Research*, **23**, 125–132.

Melzack, R., and Wall, P. (1965) *The Challenge of Pain*. Penguin, Harmondsworth.

Michelsen, D. (1978) Giving a great back rub, *American Journal of Nursing*, **78**, 1197–1199.

Montagu, M. (1978) *Touching the Human Significance of the Skin*. Columbia University Press, New York.

Moore, K., and Altmaier, E. (1981) Stress innoculation training with cancer patients, *Cancer Nursing*, **4** (10), 389–393.

Munro, S., and Mount, B. (1978) Music therapy in palliative care, *CMA*

Journal, **119** (4), 1029–1035.

Nordshow, M., and Bierman, W. (1962) The influence of manual massage on muscle relaxation: Effect on trunk flexion, *Journal of American Physical Therapy Association*, **42** (10), 653–657.

Parriott, S. (1969) Music as therapy, *American Journal of Nursing*, **69** (8), 1723–1726.

Quinn, J. (1984) Therapeutic touch as energy exchange: Testing the theory, *Advances in Nursing Science*, January, 42–48.

Sachett, J., and Fitzgerald, J. (1980) Music in hospitals, *Nursing Times*, October 16, 1845–1848.

Saunders, C. (1980) Caring to the end, *Nursing Mirror*, September 4, 52–53.

Scull, C. (1945) Massage — physiologic basis, *Arch. Phys. Med.*, **26**, 159–167.

Sims, S. (1986) Slow stroke back massage for cancer patients, Occasional Paper, *Nursing Times*, **82** (13), 47–50.

Smith, D. (1982) Guided imagination as an intervention in hopelessness, *Journal of Psychiatric Nursing Mental Health Services*, **20**, 29–32.

Snyder, M. (1985) *Independent Nursing Interventions*, Wiley, New York.

Sodergren, K. (1985) Guided imagery. In Snyder, M., *Independent Nursing Interventions*. Wiley, New York.

Tamez, E., Moor, M., and Brown, P. (1978) Relaxation training as a nursing intervention versus pro re nata medication, *Nursing Research*, **27** (3), 160–165.

Temple, K. (1967) The back rub, *American Journal of Nursing*, **67**, 2102–2103.

Vega, R. (1975) Shiatsu: A pressure technique, *Physical Therapy*, **55** (4), 381–382.

Watson, W. (1975) The meaning of touch: Geriatric nursing, *Journal of Communication*, Summer, 104–112.

Weil, G., and Goldfried, M. (1973) Treatment of insomnia in an eleven year old child through self relaxation, *Behavioural Therapy*, **4**, 282–284.

Wells, N. (1982) The effect of relaxation on post-operative muscle tension and pain, *Nursing Research*, **31** (4), 236–238.

Woody, R. (1980) *The Use of Massage in Facilitating Holistic Health*. Charles C. Thomas, Illinois.

Zeller-Dobbs, B. (1985) Alternative health approaches. Oncology nursing 6, *Nursing Mirror*, **160** (9), 41–42.

Part 6   Coordination of Care

Nursing Issues and Research in Terminal Care
Edited by J. Wilson-Barnett and J. Raiman
© 1988 John Wiley & Sons Ltd.

CHAPTER 9

The Role of the Nurse in Family Support

ANN NASH

The dying and death of a person will have a devastating effect on the members of that person's family, and will enforce unwanted rearrangement of relationships on them, both before and after the death.

The concept of family suggests a relatively permanent group of people, linked by love or obligation, caring or commitment, sometimes by line of descent. But here, family will be considered in wider terms, and include extended families where they exist, neighbour and close friend groups, and homosexual relationships of permanent value.

It is not within the remit of this writer to comment on family relationships and their complexities. It is sufficient to acknowledge potential or real problem relationships and to accept their effect on the nurse's role in support. It is also not the intention of this author to discuss the available material written about the nurse's role in patient support, and there is much in this area which, at some point, takes the family into account. I wish to concentrate on the research which looks to the family as a group which includes a dying patient, to explore the effect of that patient's dying on the family group, and the role of the nurse in that changing relationship. Except in two important instances, comments are confined to nursing research, some of which provides a fascinating insight into the nurse's role in this complex situation.

Before considering the nurse's role, specific differences should be mentioned. The nurse in hospital will have a very different role from the health visitor, but the role of the Macmillan nurse will complement and overlap that of the district nurse and health visitor. No attempts to clarify the role of the nurse in different situations will be made, but simply to explore those components of the nurse's role in family support which can usefully be applied in any situation.

Within the role of the nurse there will be many elements. There will be a role for expert, adviser, decision-maker, teacher, enabler. It can be expected that families will demand some or all such elements from time to time. The nurse's role must include the ability to balance and juggle such elements according to the needs of each family situation, and the available research enables the nurse to pursue the effects of action on outcome.

Support of the family is sometimes confused with that protective urge to take over, take control, encouraged by the family's expectations of the role. It is always much more difficult to allow the struggle and the suffering, to journey alongside and to reinforce the family in that struggle.

Scott (1985), in the Conference on Care of the Dying at Central Hall, Westminster in November 1985, acknowledged the role of the family in caring for dying patients and their importance overall in planning care and use of resources. Without this important resource, and our support of it as a resource, more dying patients would spend longer in hospital beds, separated from the family.

> ... 'helplessness' — that state which says 'I cannot help, I am useless' — is that ... natural or has it been induced by the way we have replaced the personal with the professional? ... we might discover old metaphors re-cast as we begin to talk about dying again in terms of a journey — as we begin to acknowledge the dying person as 'leader' — and recognize that our professional invitation on that journey is to be, along with others, both personal and professional 'companions'. Perhaps we shall learn that there is no prescription for a good death — only the dignity which allows the dying person to mark the route and to choose the pace and give us the privilege of enabling them to take that final step in acceptance and peace.

At the same conference, Wilkes (1985) said:

> ... Yet it has been confirmed that most dying patients are admitted to die in an institution more often because of the needs of the relatives than because of the needs of the patient. The family is

the unit of care that looks after most of the dying most of the time and deserves admiration and support ...

Professor Wilkes (1986) recently circulated health authorities and others with copies of a monograph based on a research project by the Trent Regional Health Authority which republishes some of the findings and interviews from 262 deaths to gather an overall picture typical of terminal illness both in hospital and at home and to review the problems revealed.

The book is entitled *A Source Book of Terminal Care* (1986), and presents a picture of routine terminal care as seen by the relatives, allowing them to speak for themselves in the sections by newly bereaved relatives. These are the comments which challenge the commonly held belief that relatives are cared for too, are always involved in care and decision-making. They present a picture of confusion, isolation and separateness from their dying relative, and their reliance on the professional carer to take control and give necessary care. This is not support of family, as it effectively removes them from their role. This is Scott's (1985) induced helplessness, which surely will lead to the family feeling unable to continue caring.

> ... a quarter of the caring relatives were over 70 years of age and the lack of support, confidence and vigour was a more important factor in leading to admission than the physical problems of the patient ... (Scott, 1985)

A similar report in the Bolton Health Authority (1986), undertaken by the Community Health Council, confirms the importance of the family in caring, and the acceptance that family support will enable the family unit to function usefully. The report highlighted the need for information, to enable the family to function, and for continued support in bereavement.

> ... The effects of not providing the main lay carer with adequate information have two distinct and undeniable consequences: first it undermines the carer's desire to provide satisfactory care for their patients and secondly it lodges a guilt complex based on information gained through hindsight that may affect the lay carer for many years after the unhappy event. Undoubtedly the sooner professionals find a way to deliver adequate information to the main lay carers of terminally ill patients, the sooner the standard

of care in the community can become an achievable and desirable alternative to hospital and hospice care ...

The Community Health Council made recommendations which directly affect the nurse's role in family support and drew specific objectives for such a role.

> ... Lay carers/families of patients who are terminally ill need to have a person whom they can approach for advice on problems to do with caring, obtaining appropriate equipment (when required), obtaining grants, benefits and other financial support they may need to continue caring, and with obtaining access to specialised services, for example the night nursing service and Macmillan nurses ...

Some, not all, of these issues are explored in the available nursing research, much of which concentrates on the patient in some isolation. There is, however, a number of useful and thought-provoking papers which have challenged thinking and may provide a useful base from which to explore further. The complexities in family relationships make it difficult to draw conclusions from such research, but the previous reports indicate the need for nurses to tackle such difficulties and to take on the challenge.

It would be useful at this stage to explore the relatively new role of the specialist nurse in care of the dying, and a recent report by Ward (1985) on home care services for the terminally ill details statistical information supplied by the home care teams of nine services, four of which were based at an inpatient hospice.

The majority of patients (52 per cent) lived with one other person — most commonly his or her spouse. Twenty-two per cent lived alone and the remainder with one or more other adults. Eleven per cent of the households contained one or more children. The report isolates information about the families concerned over a period of one year, with a large sample of 1094 patients.

Reasons for referral to the services include emotional support for family, advice on family management of patient care, social and financial problems, and families physically unable to cope with patient care. Comprehensive tables of recorded patient and family details present a useful picture of the home care nurse (Macmillan nurse) role with the family. The study also shows the reality of some of the problem areas for nurses in this specialty, in too large caseloads and overwork.

There are some interesting quotes from nurses about their perception of their role:

> ... support and advice ... acting as liaison ... with as much support as the family needs ... lifting of fear ... in the patient and his family ...

It is evident, however, that there is some danger of the nurse losing sight of the role due to overwork, overcommitment, and overinvolvement without sufficient support, and this perhaps is the basis of so many of the comments which should be made about the need for good assessment and evaluation.

The same dangers exist, then, in this specialist role as in the role of all nurses in family support. It is easier to take over than to allow close discussion with the family which will permit them to make decisions and make mistakes. This allows a level of involvement, and thus vulnerability, by the nurse which is frowned upon by some. It is true to say that, as is obvious from this very comprehensive report, nurses begin to lose sight of their objectives if badly supported, badly monitored, and not held accountable for decision-making, including their awareness of their involvement and vulnerability. It would be wrong to assume from this report that such nurses are not able to function well, simply that we must learn the lesson of specialization in an area of care which is so personal, and provide for it in our management of the role.

Before leaving the specialist role, it would be difficult not to mention the very new report by Lunt and Yardley (1986) not yet published but already causing ripples amongst specialist nurse teams. A survey of home care teams and hospital support teams for the terminally ill was carried out by the Cancer Care Research Unit on behalf of the National Society for Cancer Relief during 1985/1986. Forty-five services agreed to take part in the study; these ranged from independent hospices to NHS-based teams. The study is too large to discuss in detail, but the report contains useful recommendations, particularly for new services, based in part on the problem areas identified.

Many lessons should be learned by those now observing the growth of this specialist nurse role which can be applied to all nurses. We would all acknowledge our own vulnerability when caring for patients and families with whom we identify closely, and we can all recall the feeling (implied or real) of professional failure at that very vulnerability. Caring for dying patients and families learning such hard lessons of coping brings us face to face with personal loss, past or potential, and it is at this point that we begin to make decisions about our role.

It is difficult to remain objective in such situations, and may be threatening to objectively assess and evaluate nursing intervention. The picture is further clouded by the expectations of the patient, and particularly of the carer, about the nurse's role.

This difficulty with the expectations of the carers has been explored in two studies which indicate the problem for nurses. Skorupka and Bohnet (1982) asked the family members of patients being cared for in a home care hospice setting, which nursing behaviours they perceived as most helpful.

Whilst defining one of the prime considerations of hospice care to be 'to allow patient and family to remain in control and participate in planning and decision-making', this small study suggests that families identify the most helpful behaviours to be those which provide directly for the patient and not for the carer. The researchers confirmed that families rarely expect professional carers to give care to any other than the patient, and that the nurse's approach should be concrete, supportive and somewhat task orientated, meeting the caregiver's priority for patient physical care and support. The implication is that family support will occur by diffusion, but perhaps this is simply the easiest option.

Welch (1981) carried out a similar, much larger study, again asking family members to identify those interventions which were most helpful. Consistent strong agreement was noted on those statements which were linked to direct delivery of physical care to the patient by the nurse, the family member indicating that high standards and reliability were of great concern. Welch suggests that this concern may have some bearing on the reluctance of family members to leave the patient and their insistence on the bedside vigil. Family members also suggested the importance of being present while such care was delivered, and confirmed their belief that such care was best given by the nurses.

It is more difficult and certainly more time-consuming to assist and support the family member or carer in caring, in giving care, than to give such care directly. Perhaps there is also a certain reluctance on our part to relinquish those tasks which are comfortably 'nursing' in favour of an enabling, supportive role.

These studies, then, raise many important issues regarding the perceived role of the nurse in family support. The expectation of the family members is that the nurse will deliver high standards of care to the patient and this expectation is reinforced by the nurse. The family's reliance on the nurse for the delivery of such care is interesting, for she undoubtedly has the skills necessary and is able to meet their expectations, although Welch (1981) implies their trust in that is incomplete. It is possible, however, that the nurse does not encourage the family's involvement in care to such an extent that her own role must change. And yet the family can, given the necessary information and skills, achieve high, or even higher, standards of care. It is their belief that they cannot, or should not, which is maintained. This view is supported in a study by Bloomfield (1986) which explores the reaction of the family members to the suggestion of planned involvement of relatives for patients in an institutional setting.

These were patients suffering from senile dementia, admitted to hospital because the relatives could no longer cope. The aim of the study was to ask whether such planned involvement could improve the quality of life for those patients, and to question to what extent staff should concern themselves with relatives' problems in that involvement.

The relatives expressed guilt at having to have the patient admitted and stated their wish to be involved, to the extent of offering such care to other patients in the ward who did not have family members visiting. All those interviewed were prepared to be involved in delivering care, under the guidance of nursing staff. Whilst accepting the admission as necessary, their involvement in care would help the inevitable feelings of guilt about 'getting rid' of the patient.

The reactions of the nursing staff were, in general, supportive of the involvement of relatives in direct patient care and decision-making. However, 22 per cent of the nurses were against the involvement of relatives in identifying and meeting patients' needs.

This study is considered for several reasons. It confirms the view that the concept of involvement of family in institutions in caring is not always acceptable to nurses. It is also important that our exploration of the delivery of 'good' terminal care is not dependent on studies about cancer patients and their families. Long-stay wards and areas such as that described by Bloomfield are often neglected by those working towards improving standards of care for dying patients and their families. Such areas should be among those benefiting from the work done by hospices and specialist teams, and should be in the forefront of such work.

A report by Doscher (1986) of a new unit, the Co-operative Care Unit of New York University Medical Center, which aims to transfer responsibility from the professional carers to the patient and family, suggests a radical, cost-effective way of caring. The unit is based on education of patient and family carer, to enable them to perform necessary nursing and caring tasks and to become independent of the institution. This is achieved by sharing decision-making, and by enabling the family to take such responsibility. The report suggests that the unit achieves the opposite of the 'induced helplessness' discussed earlier, and further studies are in progress to evaluate the effect of the unit on prevention of readmission and to assess patient and family satisfaction.

In terms of favourable costings and effective caregiving, this model should lend itself to many areas of care, particularly those areas where early discharge is desirable.

So much care is given by nurses to patients and families without useful assessment of need. It is assumed that, as soon as a person becomes a 'patient', nurses swing into action in a fiercely stereotyped 'nursing' role which does not necessarily ask what it is that the nurse should or could do that someone else might do better or more appropriately.

Studies of family crisis have produced a framework within which the nurse can assess the factors affecting the family's ability to cope. MacVicar and Archbold (1976) suggest a model which enables nurses to break down the factors and provides the nurse with a guide towards approaching this complex area.

Lewis (1983), accepting that it is the family, not just the cancer patient, who experiences the stress associated with the disease, attempts to measure the impact on the family and the effect of services on the family.

Assessment may be influenced by fallacies in reasoning about family-directed services, and this may affect action by the nurse. Lewis explores several fallacies which may affect the role of the nurse. Family function is made complex by variables such as cultural background, past history and other factors. It is dangerous, then, to simplify the reasons for disequilibrium. Families need to work through grief in their own time, and Lewis suggests that intervention can be unwarranted if the family is not ready. It is sometimes more useful to be alongside and to adopt a stance of 'non-action', and not try to ameliorate the pain. In this way, the nurse affirms the family's worth rather than trying to change the way it functions. This is a difficult role; it is more comfortable to try to 'make it better'. This paper enables the nurse to view the family's needs in its own terms and to avoid some of the pitfalls of trying too hard.

Suggestion has been made that patient-centred issues will affect the family by 'diffusion', and that such patient-centred care will inevitably lead to family support, a view supported and reinforced by the family members themselves. Lewis suggests that this approach is unrealistic, that such families may assume that the carer is only interested in the patient, and that the real concerns and distress of the family would be missed. Family assessment is difficult, time-consuming and confusing, and it is much easier to direct care at the patient, seeing the family as a necessary, if irritating, adjunct. It is not many years since patients and families were physically separated during hospital admissions, and allowed an hour or two's visit during the evening. Most of us (nurses) grew up through and with this system, unquestioning of its effect on the family. We have not moved enough steps away from it to take on change sufficiently to enable us to really give family-centred care.

Dying, however, is a personal issue. It is something which will happen to us all, and has probably already happened to someone we held dear. Our experience of the personal issue of dying and of personal loss will inevitably affect our response. It is therefore with a great deal of emotional 'baggage' that we approach this family's distress.

I was unprepared for my first contact with such distress and was hurt and embarrassed by it. It is upsetting today to hear that comment repeated by students in training around the country. Surely we learned by our own distress to prepare our students better and give them ample opportunity to explore their feelings before meeting them head on? Or, by the time we reached the dizzy heights, had we forgotten how painful that experience was? It is certainly possible to place great distance between what might have been the natural reaction to pain and sharing pain with patient and family, but the price is great.

Much of my discussion with nurses about their role with such families centres around the personal issue, involvement, sometimes discouraged and sometimes seen as failure. I was interested, then, to look at studies which explored how nurses felt such involvement affected their role.

A study by MacDonald and MacNair (1986) in the Wandsworth Health Authority aims to determine district nurses' perceptions about the problems and satisfactions of caring for terminally ill patients at home. District nurses are the key to families being able to cope at home with patients who are terminally ill, and this study attempted to determine which factors affected that role. The family is acknowledged to be the major resource available in community care and the district nurse's role in enabling them to cope is well documented. Our experience suggests that dying patients wish to remain at home for as long as possible, and possibly to die there. Families who believe that nurses are the only people who can deliver good care to their dying relative will feel inadequate and may agree to hospital or hospice admission because of these expectations. What happens in the community, therefore, will set the seal on the fate of this family, and this in turn may well affect the quality of their grieving.

Shortages of staff and too high caseloads were seen to be responsible for affecting the nurse's role in family support in this study by MacDonald and MacNair, but most nurses determined other problem areas. Nurses felt generally unprepared for their role in terminal care and their ability to support such families if their training was lacking. Early referrals would improve their ability to make relationships while the patient was well, and nurses recorded much satisfaction gained from enabling relatives to cope by teaching them to nurse the patient. This sharing of skills is fundamental to the family being able to cope and there is an awareness that this ability to provide care gives relatives a tremendous sense of achievement and eventual comfort.

The district nurse's role in mobilizing other caring services was seen as important in supporting the family. Access to night-sitting services and other supportive networks affected the level of satisfaction with care given and in general nurses felt that most patients could be managed at home. The nurses, however, detailed symptoms which, in their view, would be better managed away from home, and I would be interested to pursue this area of apparent need and particularly its effect on them and their level of satisfaction.

This problem is referred to again in a study by Woodall (1986) with hospice home care patients. Reasons for admissions were predictably those where increased nursing needs exceeded family resources and, in a large percentage, where symptoms were not controlled. Our own experience reinforces the view that many terminally ill patients are admitted to hospice or hospital beds, not because the family can no longer cope, but because symptoms are uncontrolled. This leads to a situation of lack of sleep, consequent exhaustion for both patient and family, and great stress, and the reason for admission is therefore often confused. Many hospices, of course, expect to include family members in all aspects of care and to maintain the family's control while the patient is in, and perhaps we could further investigate how other units may perform in similar ways.

Baider and Porath (1981) report on nurses' experiences of terminal care on a cancer ward at Hadassah Hospital in Jerusalem, the authors working with the nurses in enabling them to explore their role with the families. The patient's family often eat and sleep on the ward. As a result, the nurses get to know not only the patient, but often the entire family very well.

A group was formed to enable the nurses to communicate their needs, to determine common experience and to explore their personal fears and feelings. New nurses attributed their feelings of insecurity in emotional situations to lack of expertise and experience, while older nurses felt unable to come to terms with emotions they judged as inappropriate in experienced nurses. Neither group was, therefore, able to share, and both felt ashamed of their feelings. Both groups thus felt alienated and alone. These feelings affected the nurses' approach to caring and their willingness to become involved. Some nurses found they could deliver 'efficient' care without becoming 'overinvolved', placing emotional distance between themselves and the families, whilst other nurses paid the price for their level of involvement with vulnerability and often took out their feelings on their family at home.

The nurses found that, by working closely with families, they identified with them and became involved in anticipatory mourning. They reported difficulty in separating their professional role from private feelings:

> I met his whole family, wife, four children, and other members of the family who came to visit. I talked with them as if they had been my own family. When there wasn't much to do on the ward, I would take the children for walks around the building or in the grounds. Afterwards, Mr P couldn't hear enough about our outing and wanted to know every detail, especially about his children.

The nurses used the group to explore their own feelings about death and their reaction to loss, so that they might feel able to approach families in a supported, realistic way.

Group sessions such as this can provide nurses with a forum in which to examine feelings and to address the 'too painful' areas of caring, making it possible to continue involvement. The sessions in the study were, unfortunately, discontinued after seven months, due to heavier workload and a need for a break from the issues faced!

Smith and Varoglu (1985) describe a qualitative study into how nurses interpreted a supportive working environment when caring for dying patients and their families, and how such an environment might affect their approach in family support. Nurses commented how much involvement the family demanded of them, according to the support and closeness of the family group, and how draining emotionally the situation could be when conflicts with the family remained unresolved.

These hospice nurses acknowledged their role in enabling families to grieve, and how difficult that role was when they had to share emotionally difficult times with them. This involvement, however, was not seen as failure but as part of their role.

These nurses, then, were aware and vocal about their need for support in such circumstances, and they did not see that need as weak or shameful. The authors suggest that the support behaviours of nurses in non-hospice units may not be so useful and this view is supported by this author's own work. Indeed, in hospice units, too, such support is not always as available as one would believe, sometimes paid lip-service to, and sometimes degenerating into a discussion about drugs and syringe pumps.

Perhaps in some instances, hospice nurses, by dealing with death on a daily basis, have been forced to face the personal issues and share them with colleagues in order to survive. While participating in support groups, as described in this study, is voluntary, there is nevertheless a need for some formal provision. Informal support, the 'open door' policy, is undoubtedly given and received and is of great value, but should never be seen as sufficient. Although much support is available, nurses in need are not always able to take it up, especially at a time of great involvement and commitment. Informal support is in addition complicated by the knowledge that co-workers are also under pressure and in need of support themselves, and nurses can be reluctant to demand support in such circumstances.

In the same way as such group experiences may provide for strength for professional carers, so nurses must explore the provision of such group support for patients and families.

Herzoff (1979) describes the group process for families of dying cancer patients and the group acceptance of emotional strength in the face of physical weakness. Such a group can provide for support for families in sharing of information and peer counselling. The role of leader is in clarification of information, redirection, cohesion and continuity. Such sharing can enable growth in families and change in the family system.

In our work with dying patients we cannot fail to be impressed by the ability of the family to grow and change in the face of loss. In our work with the families of dying children we have been privileged to observe the effect of our intervention and have tried to make some assessment of that in retrospect.

During her training in social work, Hay (1986) worked with the Dorothy House team, and became closely involved with a group of bereaved mothers who still meet months and years after the death of the child. The group allowed staff to take a critical look at the effect of professional carers on the outcome and the consequent grieving process. It is now apparent that the formation of this group before the death of the child would have been much more useful and would have enabled the nurse to plan intervention to meet the needs of each family unit. Hay's work is unpublished, but several specialist paediatric oncology units have approached the idea of groupwork for families during the child's illness and after death. However, other evaluative work than this study has not been traced.

Two studies in particular offer nurses an opportunity to examine the effect of their supportive role.

Chekryn (1984) carried out a study of couples in identified relationships where cancer had recurred; this explored the issues and the areas of need for patient and carer, particularly the carer closest to the patient. The study suggests that there must be a deliberate move towards including family members in the assessment process if the nurse is to enable them to address some of the problem areas together. Nurses must not underestimate their role in enabling such communication between family members, especially in the painful area of talking about dying and dying-related issues. The ability to enter into such discussion at this difficult time may well add to the security of the family unit, even though they must now begin to grow and adapt to the new role, and can be the greatest aid to that family to become aware of their own resources.

Giacquinta (1977), again working with cancer patients and their families, describes a model of stages and phases to understand the functioning of family members in crisis and explores the nurse's role in that functioning.

The model focuses on ten phases of family functioning within four stages: living with cancer, the living–dying interval, bereavement, and reestablishment, and describes the possibilities for nursing intervention in each.

It is accepted that the roles within the family must change during the time of caring, and that family members often must adapt to now unfamiliar roles. The nurse must facilitate such change by open communication and by fostering a sense of cooperation. Giacquinta explores in some depth the improtant role of the nurse in the prebereavement work carried out by the family. This is a difficult struggle for most nurses and this study is most helpful.

The aim of nursing intervention is towards promoting the value and strength of the family in their loss and enabling them to see the value of growth in their changing identity.

The nurse is constantly faced by the prospect of identifying her role within a given family crisis. Nothing can be surer than that each crisis, whilst having similarities with others, will demand something new and different of her. There is also no doubt that she will identify personally with each crisis, some more than others, and that this may well get in the way of assessment and effective planning of care. Good caring relationships are essential to the ability of the nurse to perform in the role the family demands. We have approached the role of adviser, information-giver, decision-maker, enabler, educator, facilitator. Each family will present a different picture to confuse the issue, and this will be further confused by tradition, locality, culture and personality.

In this chapter the family has not been defined in terms of its specific members, so as not to exclude sometimes more meaningful relationships and those of truer value than the accepted meaning of 'family'. In hospices staff commonly meet all possible combinations of the relationship spectrum, and have learned not to judge relationships by what they call themselves. Our commitment to the care of patient with AIDS requires that we move ever deeper into our feelings about what constitutes 'family' and the effect of disease on that family, when that disease carries with it such a difficult history.

Nurses would all say they support families, and this chapter has attempted to question the quality of that statement and perhaps point the way to some useful work which might enable nurses to evaluate it. Support of family is so much more than it seems, especially when that family is not quite what we would like it to be — perhaps not loving, not committed to caring, perhaps divorced, single parent or homosexual. Nurses have to learn to support the unit that exists, and not some vision of family embedded in our own view of life.

References

Baider, L. and Porath, S. (1981) Uncovering fear: group experience of nurses in a cancer ward. *International Journal of Nursing Studies*, **18**, 47–52.
Bloomfield, K. (1986) Ask the family, *Nursing Times*, March 12, 28–30
Bolton Health Authority (1986) *Care of the Dying in Bolton*, Bolton Community Health Council.
Chekryn, J. (1984) Cancer recurrence: Personal meaning, communication and marital adjustment, *Cancer Nursing*, December, 491–498.

Doscher, P. (1986) When the relative is the nurse, *Nursing Times*, May 28, 28–29.

Giacquinta, B. (1977) Helping families face the crisis of cancer, *American Journal of Nursing*, October, 1585–1588.

Hay, R. (1986) Group work with bereaved mothers. Unpublished.

Herzoff, N. (1979) A therapeutic group for cancer patients and their families, *Cancer Nursing, December, 469–474.*

Lewis, F. (1983) Family level services for the cancer patient: Critical distinctions, fallacies and assessment, *Cancer Nursing*, June, 193–200.

Lunt, B., and Yardley, J. (1986) A survey of home care teams and hospital support teams for the terminally ill. University of Southampton and National Society for Cancer Relief.

MacDonald, L. and MacNair, R. (1986) Your views on terminal care, *Journal of District Nursing*, March, 11–14.

MacVicar, M., and Archbold, P. (1976) A framework for family assessment in chronic illness, *Nursing Forum*, **15** (2), 180–194.

Scott, T. (1985) National Association of Health Authorities. Conference on Care for the Dying. DHSS, HMSO, London.

Skorupka, P., and Bohnet, N. (1982) Primary care givers' perceptions of nursing behaviours that best meet their needs in a home care hospice setting, *Cancer Nursing*, October, 371–374.

Smith, S., and Varoglu, G. (1985) Hospice — a supportive working environment for nurses, *Journal of Palliative Care*, **1**, 16–23.

Ward, A. (1985) *Home Care Services for the Terminally Ill*. A report for the Nuffield Foundation.

Welch, D. (1981) Planning nursing interventions for family members of adult cancer patients, *Cancer Nursing*, 365–370.

Wilkes, E. (1985) National Association of Health Authorities. *Conference on Care for the Dying*. DHSS, HMSO, London.

Wilkes, E. (1986) (ed.) *A Source Book of Terminal Care*. University of Sheffield Printing Unit.

Woodall, C. (1986) A family concern, *Nursing Times*, **82** (43), 31–33.

Part 7   Conclusion

Nursing Issues and Research in Terminal Care
Edited by J. Wilson-Barnett and J. Raiman
© 1988 John Wiley & Sons Ltd.

CHAPTER 10

Progress in Terminal Care Nursing

JENIFER WILSON-BARNETT

Contributions to this text reflect the enormous progress that has been made over the last decade. As a central part of terminal care, nursing has been transformed in its aims, methods and philosophy. This change has also been possible because of the close multidisciplinary approach when advances in one discipline have affected practice in another. Readers cannot fail to be impressed by the dedication of those who work in this area, but it is the wisdom of so many writers which is also evident. That blend of professional experience and scholarship evident particularly in so many Macmillan nurses prompted this book. If this text fulfils its aims some of that wisdom will be even more available for the benefit of other nurses.

Progress has been achieved in methods used in clinical care, in symptom relief, in more flexible approaches to care and in innovative nursing interventions. Chapters on pain, managing difficult problems, on bereavement support, child care, on complementary nursing interventions and the overall provision of care exploit an emerging research-based literature. However, as areas for future research all these issues are immensely challenging, and more knowledge is patently required to achieve successful outcomes for all those in need. It is especially difficult to conduct research interviews with those who are distressed; their circumstances make this seem insensitive, yet it is this type of work by people like Ann Cartwright, Barry Lunt and John Hinton which has stimulated those in the health care professions to evaluate their own efforts and extend good practice througout the service as a whole.

Work within special symptom relief teams, by hospice and district-based staff, demonstrates how crucial collaboration and coordination is. This may have been prompted by the nature of the need or by the type of staff undertaking the care. Nurses have, through their caring attitudes, earned a special authority in this area. As some of the reviews show, the Macmillan nurses in particular are generally seen as a valuable resource, not just to do things that others do not want to do but as advisers to others, as a support for the family, with expertise and personal strength. Lunt and Yardley's (1987) recent work shows just how much they are needed by the community. It is partly due to their authority that others in institutional care settings have recognized the need for more expertise in terminal care.

Nursing education is now attempting to catch up with these trends in terminal care. More awareness of previous failures to provide confidence, knowledge, therapeutic attitudes and skills has led to a much greater emphasis and preparation for terminal care in the first level of nursing education. Field and Kitson's (1986) paper reflects this acceptance. However, practical experience must also be suitable to avoid reinforcing fears of death and dying which so many people hide. It seems that higher education courses are promoting the philosophies and associated skills in nursing, and appointments such as the Macmillan Lecturer in Nursing at King's College, London, are helping in these developments. Changes within continuing nursing education, with the new advanced course in terminal nursing care (285) now established, also reflect the growing body of knowledge and greater expectations of specialist nurses.

Future Research

Social Aspects of Care

Energy devoted to improving the social environment for care of the dying has had a great impact on attitudes to death. Many individuals have been involved in one way or another with voluntary organizations, by making donations or through more personal contact with the hospice movement. People have therefore been discussing facilities or even just thinking a little bit more about their own mortality. Nursing as a product of social change has also had to reflect the wishes of families to be more involved and provide more personalized care. This requires a closer and more socially relevant service where care is given as a part of family life, reflective of customs and preferences.

Community care has always faced this challenge and when people want to die at home the carers must be supported and adequately assisted. However, this ideal has not been achieved — two-thirds of patients die in hospitals and comparisons by Lunt (1985) and Parkes (1978) demonstrate that satisfaction and symptom relief is not good enough in hospitals or for those who die at home when compared to hospice-centred care. The compromise of daycare in hospices has been advised to remedy the situation (Wilkes, 1980).

Nurses must therefore keep in touch with the wishes and feelings of all the family members and assess when certain interventions are necessary. Studies of the Macmillan nurses (Lunt and Yardley, 1987) show that they constantly aim to do this, but social and economic pressures on families and the terminal care service cause problems.

There have been several studies comparing the overall effects of different terminal care provisions and the Macmillan nursing service. But there is work that needs to be done. Descriptive studies need to:

1. Explore the social costs of home care for the family
2. Examine the factors influencing the extent of choice for the context of care
3. Analyse the economic viability of some of the independent hospices and the impact of using staff time to raise funds
4. Assess attitudes of the local population to dying in a community with an active hospice team and compare this to an area without this facility
5. Study whether children's education could be modified to encourage a less fearful attitude in later life (school nurses might be involved)

Evaluation of certain interventions is also necessary, in particular:

1. Daycare, being relatively new for most centres, should be evaluated by setting goals and measuring the extent to which these are met.
2. Involving the local community in providing voluntary support is essential as part of this movement; different strategies should be compared for their effectiveness.
3. Family members are frequently involved in care; the sensitivity and continuity of carers may result in a better outcome but this should be evaluated thoroughly and compared with the effect of other carers.

Psychological Care

Knowledge of the psychological responses to a fatal diagnosis and to dying is quite advanced, as in the field of bereavement reactions and risks. Prescriptive suggestions for care, however, are less well tested. For instance, open communication is found to promote adjustment in the specialized hospice setting and a lack of this is said to lead to far more family conflict when patients die at home. Given that experts now believe that home based and supported care is most desirable for a majority, more exploration of this field and the implications is required.

Care to help patients and families feel less emotionally distressed, to feel informed and 'in control' consists of getting to know all the significant people well, spending time in order to understand their feelings, providing information of relevance and having a plan to achieve harmony and closeness. How much do we really know about what promotes this care? Several aspects of what is described as good communication are now discussed and rehearsed by nurses. Yet do we have enough evidence, as well as confidence, that we can recognize when families desire an open approach and another visitor who wants to support them and become a close family friend? Anecdotes and surveys evaluating the Macmillan services would suggest this is so for a majority, but this is such a vital area that it deserves careful exploration.

Several areas for research seem to emerge from chapters in this book for those working in terminal care. Both descriptive studies exploring the diversity of 'problematic' responses and evaluative work testing various nursing interventions, skills and attitudes are required.

Further assessment and description of responses could include work in the following areas:

1. Systematic accounts of patients' responses and how these change and are expressed could help in preparing future nursing strategies.
2. In-depth records and studies of the incidence of those with maladaptive responses should be reviewed.
3. Analysis of communication strategies, of what patients say to different people in different contexts, is needed, as well as preparation of more teaching videos to help in cue recognition and training appropriate nursing responses.
4. Interview studies with spouses to assess their nursing needs are needed in this country, e.g. replication of Hinds' (1985) work.

5. Interview studies could be carried out to explore with bereaved family members those nursing actions which were considered helpful or unhelpful.

Evaluative studies also need to be carried out:

1. Assessment of visiting patterns would help to plan a study evaluating 'regular' *versus* 'crisis' visiting on the emotional adjustment to dying patients and their families.
2. A retrospective study with families rating psychological carers to identify good role models and behaviours.
3. Evaluation of role models/teachers in hospital ward settings using the following criteria:
    (a) Patients' satisfaction with information, support and caring attitudes of staff.
    (b) Nurses' knowledge, attitudes and time spent with dying patients and their relatives.
    (c) Communication skills of all members of the health care team.
    Such studies could compare before and after introductions of role models/teachers or across wards.

'Coping' with Dying — the Patient and the Family

This abstract term is very difficult to operationalize and study. Strategies for coping by patients, families and nurses have been reviewed in some of the preceding chapters. Ultimately positive coping is influenced by previous patterns of successful coping with earlier life experiences. Conflict, lack of support and physical distress make this even more difficult for a patient, and indeed for the spouse.

Advances in knowledge and understanding have been made by nurse researchers such as Dracup and Breu (1978) and many others, but Lazarus (1983) still admits that more research is required to understand what behaviour facilitates coping in which contexts. It is probably in this area that the experts could provide many insights and much case material and more systematic records would be helpful to promote this.

Coping with physical difficulties is also of paramount concern since patients in the terminal phase are usually symptomatic, as Twycross (1986) reports. Such progress has been made in symptom control that this knowledge needs to be applied everywhere, not just in those specialized settings. However, patients themselves often employ their own strategies (such as visualization or imaging) in conjunction with medical treatment. These may be valuable for others, and nurses can manage to teach them to others.

It is often the case that patients are the most valuable asset to others who are dying and their families. Groups have been used in other countries, e.g. Yalom and Greaves (1977), and even more contact between fellow sufferers is found to assist in adjustment (van den Borne, Pruyn and van den Heuvel, 1987). So perhaps these should also be tried and tested.

Descriptive work exploiting theoretical ideas from 'coping' psychology would be valuable; for example work could include:

1. In-depth interview studies which explore patients' coping ideas and strategies aimed to promote psychological adjustment and alleviate discomfort.
2. Systematic record-keeping by nurses involved in bereavement counselling to study the frequency of use for certain coping strategies.
3. Careful analysis of clinical problems facing nurses, i.e. discharges, incontinence, malodour, to assess their prevalence and management.
4. Assessment of need for equipment and services across health districts by family visits.
5. Interview studies with nurses to assess their own strategies for coping with this type of work.

Evaluation is also needed in order to see which methods are best in which circumstances:

1. Physical symptoms should constantly be assessed and care evaluated and compared by their incidence and the time taken to resolve such symptoms.
2. Group discussions with patients and spouses should be evaluated for their effects — possibly in a daycare setting.
3. Nursing actions in managing symptoms should be evaluated and this could be done as a field study in which Macmillan and district nurses monitor such problems.
4. Support groups for nurses, helplines and other existing arrangements should be compared for their effectiveness, stability of the team and mental health of the nurses.

Comfort Care

Children with their comforters display their need for security; adults also need extra care to tolerate this most difficult time of their life. Emotional support from a caring family or helpful nurse is fundamental to comfort, but the good or helpful nurse understands and provides the right touch, the smooth unruffled manner and the interesting diversions that are needed. Documenting details of what this consists of is extremely difficult and to some extent impossible. However, modern institutional care often fails to provide for these and other comfort measures. Whereas hospices and home care can provide comfort care, the evidence that district general hospitals cannot, unfortunately, exists (Hockley, 1983; Lunt, 1985).

Innovations for nursing have often arrived after others have used them for the healthy or in other countries. This seems to be the case in Sally Sims' Chapter 8. Massage seems to be only too obvious as a helpful and relaxing intervention. Relaxation therapy and music therapy may also help different people or all of them at different times. Their availability is obviously necessary prior to assessing their use.

Assessment of methods relies on sensitive, usable and reliable tools. Pain measurement has benefited from continuous work in this area as Jennifer Raiman showed. But for other symptoms it is somewhat limited and more research needs to be done on tools to assess both psychological and physical responses. Symptom checklists with simple scoring methods are needed for use in clinical work and research.

Descriptive work should involve both interview and observation studies:

1. In-depth interviews with specialized nurses should aim to explain what they see as comforters and what they do to ensure patients feel really cared for.
2. Spouses should also be interviewed about their experiences of providing home comforts.
3. Hospice care and environmental aspects of this need to be methodically described and compared to other clinical settings to assess how extra comforts could be introduced into hospitals.
4. Measuring tools for assessing feelings and symptoms need to be devised and those that exist need more reliability testing.

Evaluation of 'comfort' interventions should be carried out, despite the existence of so many extraneous and endogenous variables which make this so difficult.

1. Back massage should be provided by most nurses, as appropriate.
    A replication and field trial of Sims' (1986) pilot study is needed.
2. Relaxation therapy should also be evaluated for use in many
    settings by both patients, relatives and nurses.
3. Those studies replicating Simonton and Simonton's (1974) and
    other imaging techniques need to be undertaken in this country.

Coordination of Care

As the member of staff in the 'front line' or in continuous contact with
patients and relatives, the nurse should be able to accurately monitor
patients' responses to their situation and to certain treatment. To do
this knowledge of others' plan of care and relationships is important.
In the favourable hospice settings, where the ratio of nurses to patients
is 1 : 1.5, this should be expected. However, in the hospital setting,
where acute treatment and other priorities for care seem to mitigate
against such intense and continuous care, dying patients need the
attention of either a specialized palliative care nurse (Hadley and
Jones, 1980) or care teams (Hockley, 1983).

Working together in a multidisciplinary team is advised by official
working party reports (Wilkes, 1980), but this occurs with variable
success in the community settings where non-specialists are concerned
(Lunt and Yardley, 1987). All the professional skills of the district and
Macmillan nurse in relating to general practitioners and other district
staff are required to coordinate care skilfully. More action research on
seeing how this can be done in certain situations would be valuable.

One fundamental aspect of multidisciplinary care is the sharing of a
common purpose or objective for care. It seems that goal-setting is
more commonly practised in the hospice setting by doctors but is only
just being introduced for the direction of nursing care. Lunt and
Jenkins' (1983) work with nurses showed that this could be achieved
and that nurses tried hard to continue this when possible. More
collaboration on shared goal-setting would not only perhaps help
coordinate care but would provide a ready-made tool for close
evaluation of clinical care. On-going Cancer Research Campaign work
with Jones and other GPs in Exeter to evaluate use of a multidisciplinary
cooperation card for use with terminal patients is encouraging.

Several projects in this area have been carried out and Lunt and
Yardley's (1987) recent work demonstrates the many difficulties that
specialist nurses have when working in situations where they are too
isolated.

Possible projects for the future could be carried out along the following lines:

1. To assess the influence of prevailing priorities of care among general nurses and then the effects of more specific educational strategies highlighting the needs of terminal patients.
2. Patterns of multidisciplinary care should be described in different care settings to demonstrate how staff work together and to identify any barriers.
3. Different types of coordination by nurses need to be explored to identify ideal practice for purposes of further nurse education.
4. The role of the nurse in terminal care coordination needs to be explored with other staff to assess whether this is acceptable to them and question what measures should be undertaken to ensure it is feasible.

Evaluation studies also need to be done:

1. Action research on introducing methods of goal-setting might well be undertaken in hospital and community settings.
2. Study days or workshops with nurses to discuss coordination problems could be evaluated for their effectiveness in solving problems.
3. Evaluation of multidisciplinary terminal care teams is being done in several centres by local staff; a more representative evaluation in many centres may assess their effectiveness.

Future Strategies: Nursing Education and Care of the Terminally Ill

More elderly people and more patients dying of malignant disorders justifies greater effort in improving the nursing care given to the dying. Deficiencies in the present pattern of care, where over 60 per cent of people die in hospital and the majority of these die alone (Bowling and Cartwright, 1982), must be rectified. General shortages of well-trained nurses are to blame in part and this requires political recognition that nursing care and nurses deserve more resources.

Progress in both the proportion of time devoted to the subject of palliative care and the interactive methods used to educate needs to be extended in all settings. There is some early evidence that graduate courses emphasize the role of psychological care and result in greater attention being given to this by graduates (Field and Kitson, 1986). This indicates that higher-level educational preparation can help to make nurses more comfortable and willing to provide what is sadly neglected in many settings.

In summary, there is evidence that in the future:

1. First-level nursing education should emphasize care of the dying throughout courses to ensure more confidence and skill.
2. Higher-level courses are needed, continuity of such opportunities affording more integration with professional practice needs.
3. More supportive managers, workshops and group studies should be organized to sustain motivation of terminal care staff.
4. Multidisciplinary education at different levels is considered useful by many educationalists and more efforts in this direction are required.
5. Role models of good practice should be introduced into care settings that have little expertise in the field of terminal care nursing. Perhaps Macmillan nurses prepared for this role would be acceptable.

Whenever practice is examined, there are always areas where improvements can be made. However, there seem to be tremendous variations between different areas. Good practice in some areas should be shared with others needing examples and role models. This would help to integrate education and practice in terms of communication skills, psychological care and symptom management.

Goal-directed nursing would seem to be needed in many settings and reflects the present philosophy of problem-oriented care. Multidisciplinary collaboration in this would be ideal but it would also help to prioritize care for groups of patients, particularly when the curative treatments and palliative approaches both prevail, as in acute wards or primary care settings.

At the more advanced stage specialist nurses have pressed for continuing education at levels suitable for their responsibilities. Despite generally favourable evaluations of the basic ENB course, the greater demands and expectations from families in the community and the expanded knowledge in this area of care have necessitated a more advanced course. Ongoing evaluation of the two first advanced courses at St Christopher's Hospice and the Royal Marsden Hospital will help others to reflect the professional needs of nurses in this area. At this level multidisciplinary education is called for to promote collaboration.

Work in medical schools in Glasgow by Calman and in Dundee by Harden is encouraging for such initiatives.

Whether one classifies workshops or group meetings as education or support for staff, their existence is seen as invaluable by participants. There should be no doubt that all those working in this area need to feel supported, as attrition and burnout in this professional group must be alleviated (Maguire, 1985). Coping is facilitated when the individual perceives s/he is well supported. Regular meetings such as those held by the National Society for Cancer Relief for Macmillan nurses are seen in this light. Not only do likeminded people come together to exchange information and learn from each other, they also gain strength from the recognition that their work is important and difficult.

Nursing education is going through fairly radical changes. One of its major changes is in the acceptance of critical appraisal of knowledge, research and practice. There is now far less emphasis on factual learning and much more on developing the intellect to prepare for coping with future professional demands and on gaining skills which help with interpersonal relationships. All this means that methods of education are going to change. Student-led seminars, self-directed learning and skills training with video feedback for the individual's own scrutiny will exist in the future.

The five key functions seem to fit terminal care rather well. If they could become more explicit in nursing education and practice, nurses' unique contribution may be recognized by other staff, as they seemingly always have been by patients and families. Future plans should reflect increased energies directed towards nursing research, education and practice in this vital area where the community have been so proactive and supportive.

In summary:

1. Family care and a community orientation have greatest relevance in terminal care.
2. Psychological care is a special responsibility fulfilled by nurses, every one of whom needs to improve necessary skills.
3. Coping skills need to be understood and facilitated by all involved in terminal care.
4. Providing comfort is essential. Nurses must learn how to do this.
5. Teamwork and shared goals, careful assessment and evaluation should lead to greater collaboration within the health care team.

References

Bowling, A., and Cartwright, A. (1982) *Life After Death: A Study of the Elderly Widowed.* Tavistock, London.

Dracup, K.A., and Breu, C.S. (1978) Using nursing research findings to meet the needs of grieving spouses, *Nursing Research*, **27** (4), 212–216.

Field, D., and Kitson, C. (1986) Formal teaching about death and dying in UK nursing schools, *Nursing Education Today*, **6**, 270–276.

Hadley, A., and Jones, D. (1980) The care of terminally ill patients: An assessment of a new approach. Unpublished research, Department of Nursing Studies, King's College, London, April.

Hinds, C. (1985) The needs of families who care for patients with cancer at home: Are we meeting them? *Journal of Advanced Nursing*, **10**, 575–581.

Hockley, J. (1983) An investigation to identify symptoms of distress in terminally ill patients and his/her family in the general medical ward. Nursing Research Paper, City and Hackney No. 2.

Lazarus, R.S. (1983) *Psychological Stress and the Coping Process.* McGraw Hill, New York.

Lunt, B. (1985) A comparison of hospice and hospital care for terminally ill cancer patients and their families, final report. Southampton University, November.

Lunt, B., and Jenkins, J. (1983) Goal setting in terminal care: A method of recording treatment aims and priorities, *Journal of Advanced Nursing*, **8**, 495–505.

Lunt, B., and Yardley, J. (1987) *A Survey of Home Care Teams and Hospital Support Teams for the Terminally Ill.* Cancer Relief Macmillan Fund, London.

Maguire, P. (1985) Barriers to psychological care of the dying, *British Medical Journal*, **291**, 1711–1713.

Parkes, C.M. (1978) Home or hospital? Terminal care as seen by surviving spouses, *Journal of the Royal College of General Practitioners*, **28**, 19–30.

Simonton, O.C., and Simonton, S.S. (1974) Belief systems and management of the emotional aspects of malignancy, *Journal of Transpersonal Psychology*, **7**, 29–47.

Sims, S. (1986) The effect of slow stroke massage in the perceived well being of female patients receiving radiotherapy for cancer. MSc thesis, King's College, London University.

Twycross, R. (1986) Hospice care. In Spilling, R. (ed.) *Terminal Care at Home*, pp. 96–112. Oxford Medical Publications, Oxford.

Van den Borne, H.W., Pruyn, J.F.A., and van den Heuvel, J.W.A. (1987) Effects of contacts between cancer patients on their psychosocial problems, *Patient Education and Counselling*, **9**, 33–51.

Wilkes, E. (1980) Terminal care: How do we do better? *Journal of the Royal College of Physicians*, **20** (3), 216–218.

Yalom, I.D., and Greaves, C. (1977) Group therapy with the terminally ill, *American Journal of Psychiatry*, **134**, 396–400.

Index

progress in terminal care nursing
(*cont.*)
evaluation of nursing interventions 207
nursing education 211–12
nursing practice 212–13
psychological care 206–7
social aspects of care 204–5
progressive muscle relaxation 166–8
psychological care 6–8

reflexology 170, 174–5
Registered Nursing Association of Ontario 31
relaxation 86, 146, 169
techniques 165–9
rhizotomy 144

St Christopher's Hospice 25, 29
St Joseph's Hospice 29
senile dementia 191
Shiatsu 170, 174–5
sleep impairment 102–3
Society of Compassionate Friends 64, 67
Source Book of Terminal Care, A (1986) 187
spiritual care 8

squashed stomach syndrome 94, 100
stress reduction techniques 86
substance P 123–4
symptoms of terminal illness 142–3

taste changes 97, 98 (table)
Tay-Sachs disease 54
teaching needs for families 92–3
touch 169–72
transcendental meditation 86
transcutaneous nerve stimulation 145

Welch study (1981) 190–1
What to Do After a Death (DHSS) 45
widowers 38
widows 38–9
Wisconsin Brief Pain Questionnaire 150
wound healing impairment 104
cleansing 107
debridement 107–8
haemostasis 108
nutritional status 106 (fig.)
odour control 108–9

yoga 86, 147